Menstrual disorders

What does modern medical science know about menstruation? The menstrual cycle is less well understood by physicians than is commonly assumed, and medical understanding of disorders associated with the menstruum is also limited. In this study Annette and Graham Scambler challenge orthodox thinking in both society and medicine on menstruation and disorders associated with it.

They base their study on women's own experiences and accounts of menstruation and menstrual disorders, drawing on a wide range of studies including their own. They show that women are often socialized to interpret the menstruum in negative terms and as something essentially private to be contained within the female domain. Taking an unorthodox approach, the authors incorporate a discussion of how menstruation is perceived within male culture and how the perspective of the medical profession has remained discernibly patriarchal. They show the significance of this in relation to women's experiences within the family and at work. They end the book by focusing on the medicalization of menstruation and the advantages and disadvantages for women of the greater access to the sick role this development implies.

Designed mainly for health workers in practice and training, *Menstrual Disorders* challenges conventional thinking in both society and medicine on menstruation and the disorders associated with it. Its thought-provoking discussion of the complex issues will prompt both students and practitioners to rethink their approaches to menstrual phenomena.

The Experience of Illness

Series Editors: Ray Fitzpatrick and Stanton Newman

Other titles in the series

Diabetes
David Kelleher

Multiple Sclerosis
Ian Robinson

Back Pain
Michael Humphrey

Epilepsy
Graham Scambler

Breast Cancer
Lesley Fallowfield with Andrew Clark

Colitis
Michael Kelly

Menstrual disorders

Annette Scambler and
Graham Scambler

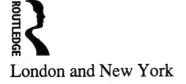

London and New York

First published in 1993
by Routledge
11 New Fetter Lane, London EC4P 4EE

Simultaneously published in the USA and Canada
by Routledge
29 West 35th Street, New York, NY 10001

Reprinted 1994

A Tavistock/Routledge publication

© 1993 Annette Scambler and Graham Scambler

Typeset in Times by NWL Editorial Services, Langport, Somerset
Printed and bound in Great Britain
by Biddles Ltd, Guildford and King's Lynn

British Library Cataloguing in Publication Data
A catalogue record for this book is available from the British Library.

Library of Congress Cataloging in Publication Data
Scambler, Annette, 1945–
    Menstrual disorders/Annette Scambler and Graham Scambler.
    p.   cm. – (The Experience of illness)
    1. Menstruation disorders – Psychological aspects.
    2. Menstruation – Psychological aspects.   3. Menstruation –
    Social aspects.   I. Scambler, Graham.   II. Title.   III. Series.
    [DNLM: 1. Menstruation Disorders – psychology. WP 550 S283m]
    RG163.S33 1993
    618.1'72'0019 – dc20
    DNLM/DLC   92–2319
    for Library of Congress   CIP

ISBN 0–415–04646–7

For Nikki, Sasha, Rebecca and Miranda

Contents

List of tables and figures   viii
Editors' preface   ix
Acknowledgements   x

1   **Medical concepts of menstrual disorders**   1

2   **A sociological perspective**   13

3   **Interpreting women's perceptions of menstruation**   26

4   **Women and help-seeking**   41

5   **Menstrual change and relationships with men**   55

6   **Menstrual change and social and work activity**   70

7   **Rethinking menstruation**   90

References   101
Name index   108
Subject index   110

Tables and figures

TABLES

1.1	Features of premenstrual tension	10
2.1	Women physicians in the NHS (UK), September 1989	14
2.2	Hospital consultants by speciality (UK), September 1989	14
3.1	Lack of understanding of the menstrual cycle	28
3.2	Menstrual symptoms most frequently defined as distressing	34
4.1	Lay consultants for general and menstrual symptoms	48
5.1	Symptoms associated with PMT in the medical literature	59
6.1	Socio-epidemiological studies on menstrual pain among adolescent girls	71
6.2	Most distressing symptoms reported during the premenstruum, by GHQ status	86
6.3	Most distressing symptoms reported during menstrual flow, by GHQ status	86
6.4	GHQ status by mean number of symptoms defined as distressing, by symptom type and by phase of menstrual cycle	87

FIGURES

1.1	Schematic description of menstruation and ovulation	3
1.2	Variations in menstrual blood loss	4
1.3	Variations in length of menstrual cycle	4
3.1	An analytic framework for women's perceptions of menstrual change	40
4.1	Local health care system	46
6.1	Menstrual pain, use of medication and absenteeism, in post-menarcheal girls aged 12, 14, 16 and 18	72

Editors' preface

Despite the fact that many women with menstrual disorders do not consult their doctor, the complaint still ranks among the ten conditions most frequent in general practice. In this book Annette and Graham Scambler first present the medical perspective on menstrual disorders, where they consider the nature of medical diagnosis and the basis for intervention. The difficulties of assessment of 'normal' menses versus 'abnormal' menses are carefully considered, and the way in which society's attitudes have impinged upon the understanding, diagnosis and treatment of menstrual disorders is discussed. The authors then present a carefully measured perspective to show how the issue of gender, which has invaded the medical perspective on menstrual disorders, creates difficulties for women in their dealings with the medical profession.

Annette and Graham Scambler are well placed to write a book on menstruation and menstrual disorders. They have been examining issues around menstrual disorders for some years and are able to draw on their own research to present women's own descriptions of their experience of menstrual disorders and their treatment. These experiences vividly illustrate the impact of this problem on women and their attempts to seek help.

This book attempts to challenge traditional concepts of menstruation and menstrual disorders through a sympathetic examination of women's experiences. The authors present the reader with a new perspective with which to view menstrual disorders. They do not, however, limit their book to a critique and an altered perspective, but in their final chapter consider an alternative way of behaving for health workers who wish to tackle this problem in a way which is sensitive to women's own perspective of the problem. In this way Annette and Graham Scambler demonstrate how an understanding of the origins of current treatment and management of menstrual disorders can lead to a new and improved approach to this common problem.

Ray Fitzpatrick and Stanton Newman, 1992

Acknowledgements

The research on which this volume builds was conducted with colleagues from the Department of General Practice at Guy's Hospital, namely, Peter Higgins, Donald Craig and Michael Curwen. We are indebted to them, although we should stress that we are alone responsible for the ideas worked out in this text. We are of course extremely grateful to the women who willingly gave their time to participate in the original study. The draft manuscript was carefully perused by the series editors, Ray Fitzpatrick and Stan Newman, and we have learned from and tried to respond to their comments.

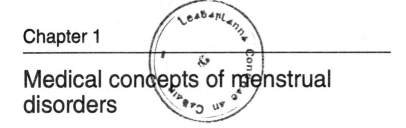

Medical concepts of menstrual disorders

The thesis that the medical perspective on menstruation and menstrual disorders is both limited and limiting will inform much of the analysis offered in this volume. It will be argued, for example, that medicine relies on applications of the concepts of normality and abnormality which are highly contentious and contestible. This first chapter, however, documents and describes rather than analyses the medical perspective. The aim is to outline the medical approach to menarche and the menstrual cycle in general, and to disorders associated with the menstruum in particular. Special attention is paid to the so-called 'premenstrual syndrome', which remains controversial within medicine as well as outside it.

MENARCHE AND THE MENSTRUAL CYCLE

The menarche is defined as the age at which the first menstrual bleed occurs. Over the past century and a half the average age of menarche has declined in modern western countries from 17 years to 13 years, the normal range now being 10 to 16 years. This decline can almost certainly be attributed to a combination of a rise in material living standards and improved and more accessible health care, since body weight at menarche seems to have remained constant throughout this period, at 45–7 kg. It has been suggested that a critical weight may need to be attained for menarche to occur (Elder 1988: 30).

The menarche occurs fairly late in puberty, which begins with a growth spurt; this is followed by the development of the secondary sex characteristics, including breast development, a widening of the hips, pubic hair, and the development of external genitalia. What the menarche indicates when it does occur is that there is sufficient activity within the ovary to have secreted some oestrogen to induce uterine development and to have caused bleeding. It does not signify fertility since, during the first two years or so, the cycles are primarily anovulatory (i.e. no ovum is discharged).

The events of the menstrual cycle are not yet well understood either in puberty or in adulthood, although there is a broad uniformity to textbook accounts which we shall follow here. The menstrual cycle in adulthood takes an average of 28 days and involves the hypothalamus, the pituitary gland, the ovaries, the endometrium and the secondary sex organs. The periodicity is inherent in the hypothalamus, which controls the cycle. The hypothalamus produces hormones, or 'chemical messengers', which act on the pituitary gland. This stimulation of the pituitary gland leads to the production of two gonadotrophic hormones: follicle stimulating hormone (FSH) and luteinizing hormone (LH). FSH brings about the development of Graafian follicles within the ovary, each follicle consisting of an ovum and surrounding cells. Approximately fifty of these follicles start to mature, but normally only one dominant follicle matures fully while the remainder retrogress. This dominant follicle enlarges under the influence of FSH and, as a result of a sudden surge of LH, ruptures and releases an ovum. Ovulation usually occurs around day 14 of the cycle.

As the dominant follicle matures and enlarges the cells surrounding the ovum produce the hormone oestrogen; and when ovulation occurs and the follicle collapses, becoming a corpus luteum or 'yellow body', the hormone progesterone is produced. These two hormones, oestrogen and progesterone, importantly affect the endometrium or lining of the womb. Oestrogen first produces thickening or proliferation of the endometrium, then progesterone produces secretions to fill the glands of the endometrium in preparation for implantation of the ovum if fertilization takes place. If fertilization does not take place, then the corpus luteum degenerates into a hyaline body known as the corpus albicans. The levels of oestrogen and progesterone fall and the endometrium is shed, appearing as blood – the process we know as menstruation. Menstruation has been described as 'the outward sign of the end of an abortive cycle and the optimistic commencement of the next' (but see chapter 2). This much-simplified account of the cycle is represented diagrammatically in Figure 1.1.

It would be misleading to leave this account of a 'normal' cycle without some comment on variation between women. Such variation has important implications, both for medical notions of disease associated with the menstruum and for women's ideas about menstrual illness. These implications will be discussed in detail in chapters 2 and 3. Here we shall merely note the extent of known variation, in relation first to menstrual blood loss, and second, to length of menstrual cycle.

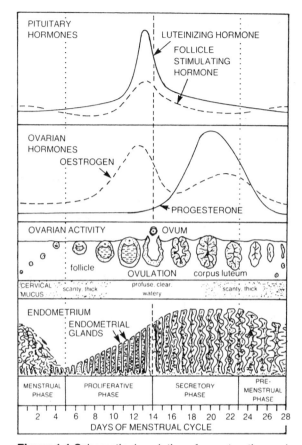

Figure 1.1 Schematic description of menstruation and ovulation

A study of several hundred women in Oxford has shown that, on average, women lose 33 ml. in menstrual blood, with 90 per cent losing less than 80 ml. and only 1 per cent 200 ml. or more; but there is considerable variation (See Figure 1.2). It is worth recording that more than 90 per cent of blood loss seems to occur within the first three days of menstruation, regardless of either the total loss or the total number of days of bleeding (average 4 or 5 days) (Anderson and McPherson 1983).

Consider also variation in cycle length. It was discovered many hundreds of years ago that the length of the menstrual cycle approximated to the phases of the moon, beginning again every 28 days. Over the succeeding centuries the 28-day menstrual cycle has become a kind of

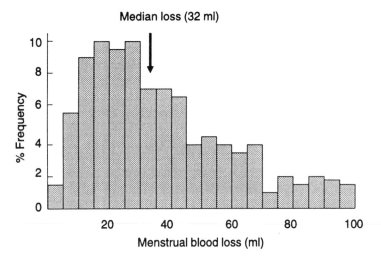

Figure 1.2 Variations in menstrual blood loss. Frequency distribution (%) of menstrual blood loss in several hundred women in Oxford before insertion of an intrauterine device.

Source: Unpublished data from J. Guillebaud, reported in Anderson and McPherson 1983

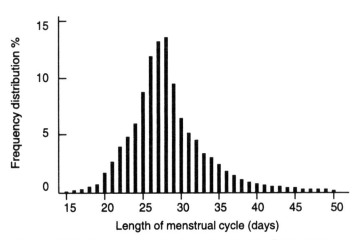

Figure 1.3 Variations in length of menstrual cycle. Frequency distribution (%) of length of menstrual cycle in days, from menarche to menopause; 31,645 menstrual cycle lengths, recorded by 656 women aged 11 to 58 years.

Source: Vollman 1977

symbol of health and normality in relation to reproductive function. Variation from the 28-day 'norm' has been and still is seen as problematic, or potentially so, by physicians and women alike. But one recent study of several hundred women from menarche to menopause has shown that, although the 28-day cycle is – just – the most common cycle length, it characterizes only 1:8 cycles (Vollman 1977). As Figure 1.3 shows, variation of cycle length is marked. This is particularly so in relation to age. Mean menstrual cycle length decreases from 35 days at age 12 to a minimum of 27 days at age 43, and increases to 52 days at age 55. Clearly the 'normality' of the 28-day cycle has to be qualified.

TYPES OF MENSTRUAL DISORDER

In the biomedical language of one recent textbook, 'menstruation depends upon an intact hypothalamic-pituitary axis, normal ovarian function, a functionally responsive uterus and an intact outflow tract, i.e. cervix and vagina. A disturbance of any one of these components may result in disordered menstrual function' (Elder 1988: 34). Three main types of disorder or, more precisely, symptoms of disorder, are commonly identified: *amenorrhoea* or absence of menstruation, *menorrhagia* or excessive menstruation, and *dysmenorrhoea* or painful menstruation. The author of the textbook cited is not alone in adding a fourth 'symptom group', *premenstrual syndrome*, but this raises special issues and will here be examined separately.

Amenorrhoea

Amenorrhoea may be apparent, primary or secondary. Apparent amenorrhoea, more appropriately termed *cryptomenorrhoea*, refers to a situation in which menstruation is occurring but the loss fails to escape from the vagina because of an obstruction, most often an 'imperforate hymen'. Primary amenorrhoea refers to a situation in which menstruation has not commenced by the age of 16 or 17; after this age it is considered less likely that it will start spontaneously. Secondary amenorrhoea refers to a situation in which menstruation ceases after it has been established for a period of months or years.

Not all physicians accept the distinction between primary and secondary amenorrhoea as useful, however. According to one text directed at general practice, for example, 'there is so much overlap in causes of primary and secondary amenorrhoea that it is not helpful to consider them as separate entities in relation to diagnosis. Instead, the differential diagnosis of amenorrhoea can be based on the main pathologies that give rise to the problem. . . . Congenital disorders usually present as primary amenorrhoea but almost all causes of secondary amenorrhoea can present as primary if they present before the age of 16 years' (Anderson and McPherson 1983: 32).

Primary amenorrhoea may be due to a variety of causes, frequently interrelated, although the mechanisms are not yet well understood. In a number of girls it derives from some genetic abnormality (e.g. failure of the uterus, vagina or ovaries to develop). In others it is a consequence of pituitary or thyroid disorders. It was noted earlier that a critical weight has to be reached before menarche can occur. Thus primary amenorrhoea can be caused by an overly rigorous diet, or by weight loss, as in anorexia nervosa; it may also be caused by obesity, although 'the degree of obesity that delays menarche is far greater than the degree of leanness that blocks the menstrual cycle' (Weideger 1975: 90). But it may also follow some traumatic episode or life event. It is often seen, for example, in women who have just left home, like student nurses (see chapter 6).

It is worth recording that the most common cause of secondary amenorrhoea is pregnancy, a possibility sometimes overlooked by women themselves. Another physiological cause is premature menopause, which can be as early as 35. Some women develop secondary amenorrhoea after stopping oral contraceptives. For others it may be associated with general disease such as pulmonary tuberculosis or severe anaemia. But, as Anderson and McPherson claim, there is a considerable overlap in the causes of primary and secondary amenorrhoea, and most of the factors discussed in the previous paragraph – from glandular disorders to weight change to life events – are equally pertinent to a consideration of the aetiology of secondary amenorrhoea.

Reference might briefly be made here to *oligomenorrhoea*, which denotes long intervals between menstruation, which may occur only two or three times a year. The term implies bleeding following ovulation. It frequently heralds either the onset of secondary amenorrhoea or premature menopause.

In a girl suffering from primary amenorrhoea who has a normal uterus and vagina, and is chromatin positive, the diagnosis is likely to be delayed menarche. Nowadays physicians generally advise waiting, since menstruation is not established in some individuals until the age of 19 or 20, and hormones given to induce bleeding may inhibit ovulation. But if a definite cause for amenorrhoea is discovered, then the treatment is that of the cause. Since, as we have indicated, both primary and secondary amenorrhoea can have multiple causes, it will not be possible to summarize all forms of treatment here. Rather, discrete causes and treatments will be dealt with in the main body of the book as and when the need arises.

Menorrhagia

Menorrhagia refers to excessive uterine bleeding with regular menstruation. It can be distinguished from *metrorrhagia*, which means irregular or continuous bleeding from the uterus; *polymenorrhoea*, which refers to frequent and often profuse menstruation; and *epimenorrhoea*, or intermenstrual bleeding, which means uterine bleeding apart from normal menstruation (Barnes and Chamberlain 1988). Menorrhagia is difficult to assess, given the extent of variation of blood loss in the female population; and, like amenorrhoea, it can have a number of different causes.

Uterine fibroids are the commonest cause; they rarely disturb cycle length, so menstruation is regular. Other lesions of the body of the uterus, or of the cervix or ovary, can present as menorrhagia. Complications of pregnancy (e.g. abortion or ectopic pregnancy) can lead to menorrhagia, as can the presence of 'foreign bodies', such as intrauterine contraceptives, in the uterus. Certain blood disorders can cause menorrhagia. Thyroid dysfunction (i.e. hyper- or hypothyroidism) is another known cause. And there can also be psychosomatic causes, for example life events involving severe emotional shock.

In as many as half the cases of menorrhagia no cause can be found, leading physicians to refer to 'dysfunctional uterine bleeding', or, as Anderson and McPherson prefer, 'unexplained menorrhagia' (1983: 21). This seems to be particularly common soon after the menarche, before the establishment of a regular cycle, and close to the menopause.

A wide range of hormonal and non-hormonal drugs are used to reduce menstrual blood loss in women with dysfunctional uterine bleeding. If a discrete cause of menorrhagia is discovered, then the treatment is that of the cause. We shall confine ourselves here to a brief consideration of the treatment of the commonest cause, uterine fibroids. It has been estimated that one in five women develop uterine fibroids, although these are generally symptomless and undiagnosed. They rarely become malignant. They usually only cause problems in pre-menopausal women, since they seem to undergo atrophy after the menopause. They can be single or multiple and vary enormously in size. Treatment depends partly on size, partly on the degree of menstrual distress, and partly on the proximity of the menopause. If the menopause is near treatment tends to be conservative, in anticipation that the fibroids will atrophy when menstruation ceases. Conservative drug therapy is also used in younger women if the fibroids are not too large. But if the uterus is considerably enlarged, or there is associated pain, then surgery may be required: myomectomy if the woman wishes to preserve her fertility, or hysterectomy if not.

Mention should also be made here of the diagnostic and therapeutic role of uterine curettage (D and C) in women with menorrhagia. Traditionally, D and Cs have been much favoured by gynaecologists. However, their value as therapeutic interventions has been called into question of late. Measurement of menstrual blood loss suggests there is no long-term benefit for women with menorrhagia. There is uncertainty also about its diagnostic role, especially in women under 35. Its main value would seem to be as a screening procedure for endometrial cancer, which is rare in younger women. Vessey and his colleagues (1979) have calculated that, taking all women under 35 in Scotland, only two endometrial cancers would be expected to be present in one year, and three to four thousand D and Cs would have to be done at the current rate to identify the two cases. Not surprisingly perhaps, increasing use is being made of alternative out-patient techniques for sampling the endometrium.

Nor would the D and C seem to be a very effective screening device for older women. Analysis of over a thousand D and Cs in Oxford in 1973 showed that all endometrial carcinomas diagnosed at curettage had presented clinically with post-menopausal bleeding (MacKenzie and Bibby 1978). Since endometrial cancer rises markedly in older women, however, curettage may still be needed to exclude malignancy in women with menorrhagia who are over 40 (Anderson and McPherson, 1983).

Dysmenorrhoea

The word 'dysmenorrhoea', deriving from the Greek word meaning 'difficult monthly flow', refers to painful menstruation. It occurs in three main forms: primary (sometimes termed 'spasmodic' or 'intrinsic') dysmenorrhoea; secondary (sometimes termed 'congestive' or 'acquired') dysmenorrhoea; and membranous dysmenorrhoea. Primary dysmenorrhoea is a common complaint. Barnes and Chamberlain write,

> Most normal women experience discomfort at the onset of menstruation, but in dysmenorrhoea pain is severe during the first hours or days of the periods; it may be continuous or spasmodic, like colic; it is often accompanied by vomiting, fainting, headaches and malaise. Pain is felt in the pelvis and lower back and may radiate to the

legs. It does not begin at the onset of menstruation when the cycles are often anovular, and it is commonest in single women or infertile married women. It tends to lessen after 25 and to disappear after 30.

(1988: 109)

Secondary dysmenorrhoea is rare before 25 and uncommon before 30. Pain usually starts three or four days before menstruation and may either be relieved or get worse when bleeding commences. It is felt in the pelvis and back and is made worse by exertion. Symptoms such as menorrhagia, sterility and dyspareunia may also be present.

The aetiology of primary dysmenorrhoea remains uncertain. There is rarely any pathological cause. One possibility is that the pain may be caused by ischaemia resulting from the powerful contractions of the uterine muscle that occur during the first days of menstruation. Secondary dysmenorrhoea does not occur without a pathological cause. The most common causes are pelvic inflammatory disease, endometriosis, fibroids and the presence of an intrauterine contraceptive device.

Treatment of primary dysmenorrhoea ranges from advice about menstrual hygiene and the use of simple analgesics to prescriptions (usually the pill) to inhibit ovulation and thus cause painless bleeding. The treatment of secondary dysmenorrhoea is aimed at the underlying cause; specific treatments will be discussed later in the text, when pertinent.

Membranous dysmenorrhoea is rare: severe pain is associated with 'the passage of all the endometrium shed at menstruation in a single "cast" ' (Barnes and Chamberlain 1988: 111). It may occur at every cycle or only occasionally. Once the cast is passed the pain is relieved and menstruation continues normally. Treatment is difficult. Oestrogen therapy and D and C may help, and in intractable cases in older women hysterectomy may be performed.

Premenstrual syndrome

The occurrence of physical and psychological changes just prior to the onset of menstruation was mentioned in the writings of Hippocratic physicians (Ricci 1950). It was not until the 1930s, however, that such changes became identified as a medical syndrome, by the American physician Frank (1931). Ever since, the ambiguous and uncertain concept of a premenstrual syndrome has caused considerable controversy within medicine as well as outside it. Consistently with our policy in this opening chapter, we shall attempt to explicate it as a medical concept, without developing any critique (see chapter 2).

Table 1.1 Features of premenstrual tension

General
1   Symptoms occur in the 1–14 days before menstruation begins.
2   After the start of menstrual bleeding the woman feels well.
3   The combination of changes occurs regularly: frequently or in every cycle.
4   PMT causes the woman distress and may cause other problems in her life.

Symptoms

Psychological changes	*Physical changes*
Depression or feeling 'low'	Breast tenderness
Anxiety	Swelling or bloated feelings
Tiredness or lethargy	Puffiness of abdomen, face, or
Tension or unease	fingers
Irritability	Weight gain
Aggressiveness	Headaches
Clumsiness or poor coordination	Appetite changes, carbohydrate
Difficulty in concentrating	cravings
Feeling less interested in sex	Acne or other skin rashes
or feeling more sexual	Constipation or diarrhoea
	Needing more or less sleep than
	usual
	Difficulty in getting to sleep
	Stiffness in muscles or joints
	General aches and pains
	Abdominal pain or cramps
	Exacerbation of epilepsy, migraines,
	asthma, rhinitis, urticaria.

Source: Sanders 1983

The medical concept of premenstrual syndrome refers to 'a collection of differing signs and symptoms which occur only in the premenstruum, i.e. after ovulation, and is relieved by menstruation' (Elder 1988: 41). The most common symptoms include depression, irritability, swollen or bloated feelings, breast tenderness and headache, although, as indicated in Table 1.1, a number of other psychological and physical changes may occur (Sanders 1983). The symptoms tend to come on 7 to 10 days premenstrually, after the luteal phase is established. In its more severe forms premenstrual syndrome is experienced most frequently in women between the ages of 30 and 40.

There are several competing theories about the aetiology of premenstrual syndrome. It has been variously attributed, for example, to oestrogen–progesterone imbalance; to fluid retention due to raised aldosterone levels in the luteal phase; to a deficiency in vitamin B6, pyridoxine; to hypoglycaemia; and to combinations of psychosocial and personality factors. Some cling obstinately to the notion that it essentially reflects a 'neurotic' personality. None of these theories has been substantiated.

According to Elder (1988: 41), treatment for premenstrual syndrome is 'largely empirical and is frequently no better than the average placebo response rate of 40%'. It is a matter of trial and error. Treatments used may be general or symptomatic. General treatments include the contraceptive pill, to inhibit ovulation; vaginal or rectal progesterone or oral synthetic progestogens; alteration of prostaglandin levels; or dietary changes, such as increasing intake of vegetable fats and vitamins. Symptomatic treatments include pyridoxine or the benzodiazepines for mood changes; bromocriptine for breast tenderness; and diuretics for feelings of bloatedness. Modern textbooks frequently stress, however, that reassurance and support may be the most important components of therapy.

PROBLEMS CONCERNING THE EPIDEMIOLOGY OF MENSTRUAL DISORDERS

There are two main sources for data on the rates of menstrual problems in the community. The first derives from consultations with general practitioners. Menstrual disorders rank amongst the ten conditions most often seen in general practice. Fry (1979) discovered the annual consulting rate for these disorders in a practice of 2,500 to be 68, with the following breakdown: 14 consulting with irregular menses, 19 with amenorrhoea or 'scanty menses', 14 with menorrhagia or frequent menses, 10 with dysmenorrhoea, and 11 with other menstrual disorders. In another general practice study, Richards (1979) found that 7 per cent of women between the ages of 15 and 50 had consulted with menorrhagia, about half of whom left with a diagnosis of dysfunctional uterine bleeding or unexplained menorrhagia. He also reported that 14 per cent of women in the same age-range had presented with a primary complaint of dysmenorrhoea.

These figures are difficult to interpret because it is abundantly clear that not all women with menstrual disorders consult their general practitioners. Nor can this interpretative quandary be easily resolved by reference to the second main source of information on menstrual problems, namely, surveys involving random samples of women in the community. This is because such surveys elicit data not on physician-defined menstrual disorders but on self-reported menstrual symptoms or distress. Reference might reasonably be made here both to the conventional distinction between medical concepts of *disease* and lay concepts of *illness*, and to the fact that there is often a poor correspondence between the two. But this distinction, although useful, does less than justice to the complexity of the phenomena under study.

Consider again, for example, excessive blood loss or menorrhagia. Note was made earlier of the considerable variation of blood loss among women. It is interesting that the medical diagnosis of menorrhagia, commonly followed by various forms of drug therapy and sometimes even surgery, is likely to be contingent upon women's subjective assessment of blood loss. 'Although objective measurement of blood loss can be made, in clinical practice this is never done, and it remains a research tool' (Anderson and McPherson 1983: 21). Yet it is known that neither women's own assessments, the number of days of menstruation, nor the number of sanitary pads or tampons used correlate with measured blood loss. Questions inevitably arise, therefore, about the rationality of diagnostic concepts like menorrhagia.

In chapter 2 we examine the rationality or irrationality of medical diagnoses and interventions in relation to menstrual disorders generally, with special reference to issues of gender. And in chapter 3 we discuss the concepts of menstruation and menstrual problems found in lay culture. Particular attention is paid to the effects of such concepts on women's definitions of what is normal and what is abnormal, and to psycho-social influences on their recognition and responses to menstrual symptoms or distress, including the seeking of professional medical help.

Chapter 2

A sociological perspective

In this chapter a sociological rather than a medical perspective on menstruation is outlined. It will be argued that the medical perspective summarized in chapter 1 is vulnerable to criticism on at least two important counts: first, whilst its advocates generally assert or assume it has legitimacy because of its foundations in science, these foundations are in fact extremely shaky; and second, medicine, like all other major social institutions in patriarchal societies, reflects patriarchal values in both its theory and its practice. The medical perspective on menstruation and menstrual disorders, then, is neither wholly scientific nor wholly neutral in relation to social conventions or mores. This is *not* to say, of course, either that physicians enjoy no autonomy at all or that they are collectively involved in some kind of conspiracy against women.

The opening section of this chapter provides a brief historical overview of medicine's treatment of women, the purpose of which is to demonstrate how, typically in the name or rhetoric of science, it has advantaged men and disadvantaged women.

MALE PHYSICIANS AND FEMALE PATIENTS

Historians have shown that healing was for centuries mainly the work of women (Stacey 1988). Thus Ehrenreich and English (1974a: 19) write,

> Women have always been healers. They were the unlicensed doctors and anatomists of western history. They were abortionists, doctors and counsellors. They were pharmacists, cultivating herbs and exchanging the secrets of their uses. They were midwives travelling from home to home and village to village. For centuries women were doctors without degrees.

Whilst women have of course continued to engage in health work, paid

Table 2.1 Women physicians in the NHS (UK), September 1989

	Total	Male	Female	Female %
Hospital medicine (*total*)	57,968	42,578	15,390	26.5
Consultant	18,449	15,687	2,762	15.0
Staff grade	33	25	8	24.2
Associate specialist	1,107	630	477	43.1
Senior Registrar	3,969	2,888	1,081	27.2
Registrar	7,754	5,901	1,853	23.9
Senior House Officer	12,999	8,189	4,810	37.0
House Officer	3,805	2,151	1,654	43.5
Other staff	23	17	6	26.1
Hospital practitioner	948	863	85	9.0
Paragraph 94 appointment	8,881	6,227	2,654	29.9
Public health medicine and community health	7,111	2,781	4,330	60.9
General practice (*total*)	34,305	25,793	8,512	24.8
Principals	31,744	24,514	7,230	22.8
Trainees	2,291	1,180	1,111	48.5
Assistants	270	99	171	63.3
Total	99,384	71,152	28,232	28.4

Source: Department of Health 1991

Table 2.2 Hospital consultants by speciality (UK), September 1989

	Total	Male	Female	Female %
General medicine group	4,941	4,311	630	12.8
Accident and emergency	230	204	26	11.3
Surgical group	3,817	3,704	113	3.0
Obstetrics and gynaecology	1,005	888	117	11.6
Anaesthetics	2,546	2,044	502	19.7
Radiology group	1,363	1,079	284	20.8
Pathology group	1,928	1,486	442	22.9
Psychiatry group	2,369	1,762	607	25.6

Source: Department of Health 1991

(even as doctors *with* degrees) and unpaid, what is of significance here is that the emergence of modern medicine through professionalization in the nineteenth century, altogether more highly regarded, influential and lucrative than its pre-modern antecedents, saw the exclusion of women as medical practitioners. Those few women such as Elizabeth Blackwell and Elizabeth Garrett Anderson who managed to get on the Medical Register established by the British Medical Act of 1858 were exceptional and anomalous. The male opposition they met with was as vehement as it was obstinate.

It was not until the 1940s that recommendations were forthcoming that women should be admitted to the hitherto single-sex London medical schools; and not until the 1970s that restrictions on the admission of women students were outlawed by sex discrimination legislation. Even at the close of the 1980s, however, when almost 50 per cent of first-year medical school places in Britain were taken by female students, women remained underrepresented in medicine's upper echelons and in its highest status and most remunerative (i.e. through private practice and the allocation of distinction awards) specialities. Table 2.1 gives the percentage of physicians who were female in the key hospital grades, public health medicine and general practice in September 1989. Table 2.2 gives the percentage of consultant physicians who were female in the key groups of hospital specialities for the same date. The relatively low percentage figure for consultants in obstetrics and gynaecology warrants a special mention here.

The reasons for women physicians' underrepresentation among medicine's elites are complex, and not merely a function of how recently female students have been accepted into medical schools in significant numbers. The extent of 'institutional', as well as 'personal' discrimination is clear: the traditional medical curricula and career structures still largely in place were designed by men for men (Allen 1988: Department of Health 1991).

Women's belated and limited career progress within medicine is an important factor in understanding the application of the medical perspective. Shelvin, a male GP, says all that requires to be said here in referring to 'the dangers of "feminine medicine" ':

> I am only too aware that an error in treatment or an impending inquest makes me practice medicine like a frightened little old lady . . . afraid . . . afraid of making definite decisions, afraid of the potential side effects of treatment (therefore using smaller, ineffective dosages), afraid of upsetting people, afraid of complaints. I pay unnecessary

visits, give unnecessary sick notes, etc, etc. Unfortunately, I often become popular during this time, people call me a 'caring' doctor. But the caring is about the wrong things. What we should care about is our effectiveness as doctors, and 'masculine medicine' is certainly effective. In this the doctor believes in himself, makes good decisions, prescribes effective treatment unequivocatingly, fairly but flexibly. A self-actualizing doctor in a self-actualizing partnership with self-actualizing patients; the goal may be unattainable, but the direction is clear.

(1981: 107–8)

Even more significant, however, is the relevance of gender to the construction of the medical perspective. Once again, an historical approach is instructive. Consider the situation in the second half of the nineteenth century. It has been said that the medical perspective on middle-class women was characterized during this time by 'the myth of female frailty'. Moreover, this myth seemed to be supported by 'the very real cult of female hypochondria' (Ehrenreich and English 1974a). It was believed not only that women were peculiarly prone to sickness, but that their sickness somehow emanated from their reproductive systems. Leeson and Gray (1978: 88) offer the following graphic account:

> doctors found uterine and ovarian disorders behind almost every female complaint, from headaches to sore throats and indigestion. Treatments ranged from blistering the groin or thighs for diseases of the genital organs and applying leeches to the labia or breasts for amenorrhoea, to removal of the ovaries to cure 'troublesomeness, eating like a ploughman, masturbation, attempted suicide, erotic tendencies, persecution mania, simple "cussedness" and dysmenorrhoea'.

Although working-class women tended to be regarded less as sick than as 'sickening', that is, as 'dangerous and polluting' (Leeson and Gray 1978: 88), an article from an 1867 edition of the *British Medical Journal* shows that they too were subjected to fashionable diagnoses and therapies. The author draws his colleagues' attention, somewhat apologetically, to an unfortunate 'evil' apparently attendant on the widespread use of the new, ingenious and generally 'beneficial' sewing-machine. He is worth quoting at some length:

> It has fallen to my lot to meet with, at the out-patient department of the London Hospital, a large and rapidly increasing number of patients who have discarded the labour of the sempstress, and assumed the business of the machinist; and I have been for some time struck with

the similarity of symptoms which many of them present. . . . These patients for the most part complain of palpitation of the heart; of palpitation, not depending on exertion, but frequently troubling them at night, when they assume the horizontal position. They speak of severe pain in the back, the pain extending down the thighs. Their pupils are usually dilated, and not very responsive to the stimulus of light. They complain of supraorbital headache, of a feeling of giddiness, and a sensation of cobwebs floating before their eyes. The eyes have diminished lustre; and beneath the orbits the skin presents a darkened hue. They nearly all complain of great debility, and it is manifest that there is existing a mental as well as a physical hebetude, as betokened by the slowness with which questions are answered, and the statuesque manner of the patient; they frequently, after the examination of the pulse at the wrist, allow the arm to remain flexed for a short time in a semi-cataleptic condition. Leucorrhoea exists in nearly all cases.

(Down 1867: 26)

On making enquiries, Dr J. Langdon H. Down (MD Lond.) discovered that the women with 'the most marked features of disturbed health' worked with machines manufactured at a single centre, and that 'the machines were so constructed that the motion was imparted by a treadle worked by the alternate up and down movement of the legs, and were heavy in their construction, being adapted for coarse work' (1987: 26). It then struck him that there was a similarity between the symptoms presented by the machinists and those he had learned 'to connect with habits of masturbation'. He continues,

Aided by this suggestion, I was not long in discovering that the series of symptoms met with among machinists was not due to machine labour *per se*, but to immoral habits, which had been induced by the erethism which the movement of the legs evoked.

(1867: 27)

He reports that a number of women recovered their health on discontinuing the machine work, using cold affusion, resorting to outdoor exercise, and taking bromide of potassium, with salts of iron. He concludes with the words,

It is not my purpose to discuss the plan which has been proposed of interfering surgically with the integrity of the female organs. Only one case has come under my observation where operative measures had been employed, and the result in that case was not such as to lead me to expect much physical or moral good from resort thereto.

In the majority of cases where the mental power has not been shattered, physical and moral treatment is of avail. In some cases, the sudden awakening to the fact that the existence of the practice can be discovered by others, calls to their aid a resolution which breaks the chains of habit, and effects a complete cure.

(1867: 27)

With the advantage of hindsight, it is of course easy enough to discern the influence of both class and gender in the construction of the medical perspective – clearly presumed to be scientific – so imaginatively utilized by Down.

The point has been made that it was middle-class women who were portrayed by male physicians as frail and liable to sickness. Working-class women, represented by Down's machinists, were manifestly not frail; indeed, it was assumed that they were generally healthy, despite their material circumstances and moral slippages. The medical theory that served to reconcile this apparent contradiction was that it was mental rather than physical work that predisposed to sickness. 'The notion that women were destroyed by brainwork rather than manual labour could thus reinforce traditional ideas about the inferiority of women and at the same time justify the very different lifestyles of middle-class and working-class women' (Doyal and Elston 1986: 179).

Ehrenreich and English are blunt in explaining the nineteenth-century physician's attitude to middle-class women.

As a businessman, the doctor had a direct interest in a social role for women that encouraged them to be sick; as a doctor, he had an obligation to find the causes of female complaints. The result was that as a 'scientist', he ended up proposing medical theories that were actually justifications of women's social role.

(1978: 129–30)

Predictably, in the light of our earlier discussion, these 'medical theories' were cited against allowing women to practise medicine. Allegedly scientific arguments of physiology and 'previously indelicate matters such as menstruation' were cited as evidence for their exclusion. John Thorburn, Professor of Obstetrics at Manchester Medical School, declared in 1884,

This is a matter of physiology, not sentiment . . . one body and mind capable of sustained and regular hard labour, and another body and mind which for a quarter of each month is more or less sick and unfit for work.

(quoted in Leeson and Gray 1978: 95)

Thorburn was not alone in arguing that study during the 'delicate' years from 15 to 25 would lead inexorably to amenorrhoea, chlorosis, nervousness, loss of femininity, infertility, and so on. A German physician, Moebius, was less restrained in a text entitled *Concerning the Physiological and Intellectual Weakness of Women.*

> If we wish woman to fulfill the task of motherhood fully she cannot possess a masculine brain. If the feminine abilities were developed to the same degree as those of the male, her maternal organs would suffer and we should have before us a repulsive and useless hybrid.
>
> (quoted in Ehrenreich and English 1978: 131)

To what extent is western medical knowledge still informed by 'convenient' gender stereotypes towards the end of the twentieth century? There is no doubt that dramatic changes have occurred in the opportunities and experiences of women of all social classes, and correspondingly in gender stereotypes, over the last century and a half; but there is no question either that medical knowledge remains discernibly patriarchal. If women are no longer regarded as physically weak, they are certainly presented as psychologically weak. Two important themes have emerged in the literature, both of them relating to medical criteria of normality and abnormality. First, while properties and attributes associated with men feature in definitions of what is normal – and therefore good – in a person, properties and attributes associated with women feature in definitions of what is abnormal – and therefore bad – in a person. And second, the properties and attributes associated with men are intimately related to the social roles men are expected to play, while the properties and attributes associated with women are intimately related to the social roles women are expected to play. What evidence can be adduced to support these themes?

A single illustration will have to suffice here, that of mental disorder. Writers such as Chesler (1972) stimulated considerable debate by attributing a new significance to sexism and patriarchy in psychiatric practice. Research through the 1970s and 1980s has both buttressed and refined this view. Concluding her review of this research, Busfield (1988) carefully identifies certain claims which she feels now 'cannot be ignored'. The first is that historically, as medicine made its transition to a modern profession, 'women were largely excluded from positions of power and authority in the hierarchy of healers, though not from healing, curing and caring per se'. There is, therefore, what she calls 'a dimension of patriarchy' in medical practice when women are patients; this dimension of patriarchy enhances the dependency of women as patients (Busfield 1988: 533).

Her second claim is that concepts of health and illness 'are not and cannot in practice be constituted independently of gender or of femininity'. In the case of mental disorder, for example, although the categories of disorder are 'formally' constituted by psychiatrists without reference to gender, gender nevertheless enters the *de facto* construction and use of these categories. Busfield gives two reasons for this.

The first hinges on the fact that in as far as conduct deemed appropriate for men and women differs and changes over time, 'then specific categories of mental illness which define certain behaviours as pathological stand in a differential and changing relation to men's and women's behaviour'. Defining excess fear as pathological, for example, is not neutral with regard to gender in cultures in which expressions of fear are more acceptable among women than among men, 'since women are more likely to manifest all degrees of fearfulness'. Busfield continues, 'Simply by acting in ways considered more appropriate to their gender women are closer to and more in danger of being phobic than men. The same is true of depression or anxiety, since the expression of these emotions is considered more appropriate in women than in men' (1988: 533–4). She points to a study conducted by Broverman and colleagues (1970) showing that definitions of male mental health were much closer to the overall norms of adult mental health than definitions of female mental health.

The second reason why categories of mental disorder are not in practice independent of gender has to do with the perception and evaluation of male and female behaviour. If women are expected, indeed required, to act in 'feminine' ways,

> which means being more dependent, less ambitious, less aggressive, more considerate, more 'expressive' than men, then the fracturing of these expectations may be defined as pathological. Women who show more independence and ambition, or who show hostility to children or spouse may be considered disturbed. Conversely men who show fearfulness or misery, or seem lacking in confidence and independence may be considered abnormal. Hence what is treated as symptomatic is not likely to be the same for men and women.
>
> (Busfield 1988: 534–5)

The third claim enunciated by Busfield is that defining women as mentally ill not only tends to make them dependent on a male-dominated profession, but also helps to ensure that little attention is paid to 'the situational aspects of their problems'. It is predominantly women who are prescribed psychotropic drugs as palliatives for problems diagnosed as anxiety disorders, depression, phobias, or other neurotic conditions (Cooperstock 1981). Individual women, it seems, need to be changed, rather than the common and often disadvantaged situations in which they find themselves in patriarchal societies.

It has been argued that women's progress both in building their own medical careers and in debunking sexist mythologies in medical texts and practices has been slow and, although more dramatic of late, remains limited. Reflections on the more extreme state of affairs in the second half of the nineteenth century are salutary in that they arm against complacency in relation to the current status quo. As Martin puts it, 'It is difficult to see how our current scientific ideas are infused by cultural assumptions; it is easier to see how scientific ideas from the past, ideas that now seem wrong or too simple, might have been affected by cultural ideas of an earlier time' (1989: 27). Having laid the foundations, it is time now to outline a sociological critique of contemporary medical concepts of menstruation and menstrual disorders.

GENDER AND MEDICAL MODELS OF MENSTRUATION

Martin (1989) has provided a useful account, again utilizing an historical perspective, of medical metaphors of women's bodies in relation to menstruation. She notes how, from the ancient Greeks until the late eighteenth century, it was generally accepted that male and female bodies were structurally similar, if not equal. They were not equal in that it was assumed that what could be seen of men's bodies provided the pattern for what could not be seen of women's, thus women were thought to have the same genitals as men, except inside the body rather than outside. Men were also thought to possess more 'heat' than women, and therefore to approximate more closely to perfection. While men rid their bodies of impurities by sweating, women – cooler and so more imperfect – did so by menstruation. 'In fact, failure to excrete was taken as a sign of disease, and a great variety of remedies existed even into the nineteenth century specifically to re-establish menstrual flow if it stopped' (Martin 1989: 31).

During the eighteenth century, however, the assumption that male and female bodies were structurally and functionally similar came under sustained attack. A new and more expansive form of biological determinism emerged.

The assertion was that men's and women's social roles themselves were grounded in nature, by virtue of the dictates of their bodies. . . .

The doctrine of the two spheres – men as workers in the public, wage-earning sphere outside the home and women (except for the lower classes) as wives and mothers in the private, domestic sphere of kinship and morality inside the home – replaced the old hierarchy based on body heat.

(Martin 1989: 32)

Now that women were no longer 'patterned' on men, the way was clear to denigrate functions seen anew as uniquely female. This change can be discerned in nineteenth-century accounts of menstruation. Menstruation itself was reconstructed as a pathological process. Geddes and Thompson wrote,

It yet evidently lies on the borders of pathological change, as it is evidenced not only by the pain which so frequently accompanies it, and the local and constitutional disorders which so frequently arise in this connection, but by the general systemic disturbance and local histological changes of which the discharge is merely the outward expression and result.

(1890: 244)

Some accounts were more vivid. Heape and Ellis, both cited by Martin (1989: 35), provide examples. Heape wrote of the entire epithelium being torn away in menstruation, 'leaving behind a ragged wreck of tissue, torn glands, ruptured vessels, jagged edges of stroma, and masses of blood corpuscles, which it would seem hardly possible to heal satisfactorily without the aid of surgical treatment'. Ellis described women as being 'periodically wounded' in their most sensitive spot, adding that 'even in the healthiest woman, a worm however harmless and unperceived, gnaws periodically at the roots of life'. In short, whereas hitherto menstrual blood may have been judged impure, now the process of menstruation itself was perceived as a disorder.

Martin is not the first to register the fact that the images commonly conjured up to represent menstruation from the nineteenth century onwards, and still conspicuous in contemporary medical textbooks, owe much to the ways in which industrial societies are organized. More specifically, the metaphor of production is frequently invoked. Relatedly, female reproductive functions tend to be interpreted teleologically, that is, in terms of their putative purpose. Martin's characterization of the treatment of female reproductive functions and menstruation in medical textbooks is worth quoting at some length:

They see the action of progesterone and estrogen on the lining of the uterus as 'ideally suited to provide a hospitable environment for implantation and survival of the embryo' or as intended to lead to 'the monthly renewal of the tissue that will cradle [the ovum]'. As Guyston summarizes, 'The whole purpose of all these endometrial changes is to produce a highly secretory endometrium containing large amounts of stored nutrients that can provide appropriate conditions for implantation of a fertilized ovum during the latter half of the monthly cycle'. Given this teleological interpretation of the purpose of the increased amount of endometrial tissue, it should be no surprise that when a fertilized egg does not implant, these texts describe the next event in very negative terms. The fall in blood progesterone and estrogen 'deprives' the 'highly developed endometrial lining of its hormonal support', 'constriction' of blood vessels leads to a 'diminished' supply of oxygen and nutrients, and finally 'disintegration starts, the entire lining begins to slough, and the menstrual flow begins'. Blood vessels in the endometrium 'hemorrhage' and the menstrual flow 'consists of this blood mixed with the endometrial debris'. The 'loss' of hormonal stimulation causes 'necrosis' [death of tissue].

(Martin 1989: 45)

It is an imagery of catastrophic disintegration, loss and death. Martin's contention is that this representation of events in terms of 'failed production' and 'failed purpose' ('menstruation is the uterus crying for lack of a baby') has contributed to our negative view of menstruation. Other, rival and more positive, representations would fit the facts equivalently well.

It is possible to identify elements of, first, *negativity*; second, *uncertainty*; and third, *irrationality*, in the modern medical perspective on menstruation and its disorders. Indeed, these elements have substantially underpinned our discussion of the medical perspective. To illustrate this, we conclude this chapter by summing up our historical and sociological commentary in terms of four key themes.

First, it has been shown that the institution of science, whether in ancient or modern guise, is neither fully autonomous nor fully value-neutral. In other words, it is a social institution. If this is most apparent in retrospective surveys of ancient or pre-modern science, it is no less true of contemporary science.

Second, medicine, even at its most scientific, reflects and reproduces patriarchal values. The negativity in the medical perspective on menstruation to which we have alluded is to be found deep in its models and metaphors as well as in the surface attitudes of its practitioners. But this is not only a reflection of its embeddedness in a patriarchal culture. Medicine also serves to legitimate and reproduce that culture. Sometimes it does so in response to third-party influence, usually the state, for example, in medicalizing or de-medicalizing menstruation according to the need for women workers (see chapter 6). And sometimes it does so unashamedly on its own account, for example, in fabricating menstrual problems in line with 'folk wisdom' to help prevent women becoming physicians ('they were seeking to use that wisdom to reinforce and shore up male privilege in the face of threats to it from the women's movement' (Sayers 1982: 116). While Laws (1990) is probably right to suggest that 'male' medicine owes more to 'male' culture than vice versa, it is a relationship that should properly be understood as dialectical.

Third, menstruation is a prime candidate for further medicalization. The extent to which this occurs will depend on many factors, but menstruation's candidature owes much to continuing medical uncertainty about the menstrual cycle and putative disorders associated with it (Laws 1990).This uncertainty gives generalist and specialist physicians considerable latitude in diagnosing and treating disorders such as amenorrhoea, menorrhagia, dysmenorrhoea and premenstrual syndrome. Medical irrationality in this context is a function of the already increasing medicalization of menstruation against a background of uncertainty. The lack of clear criteria enabling differentiation between 'normal' and 'abnormal' menstrual phenomena is of fundamental significance. Almost any presenting menstrual problem couched in an appropriate vocabulary of distress could *potentially* attract a diagnosis of menstrual disorder, quite independent of knowledge of aetiology or capacity for curative or palliative intervention.

And fourth, women typically find themselves in a 'catch 22' situation in their dealings with the medical profession over menstruation and menstrual disorders. (This is equally true of their dealings with many other institutions in a patriarchal society.) Moreover, this is an issue of increasing salience in view of recent tendencies to further medicalize the menses. There are a number of contradictions or unresolved tensions within the medical perspective on menstruation, not least because, as we have seen, it is an amalgam of 'male' science and 'male' folk wisdom. One tension, for example, is between an acknowledgement that menstruation is normal and natural for women and a (sometimes evangelical) willingness to define as pathological and to treat almost any of its manifestations perceived by women as distressing. For women to pursue medical treatment on the scale at which it is increasingly available would seem to be to affirm that what is biologically normal is socially unacceptable.

Two important riders ought to be added before the issues addressed in this chapter are explored in the contexts of women's own experiences. The first is that, for all our emphasis on what has been called the 'social construction of menstruation', it needs to be acknowledged unambiguously 'that biology [menstruation, in this case] does have real effects on women's lives and that these effects are not to be dismissed as merely the result of the ideas that societies entertain about it' (Sayers 1982: 124). And the second is that it is not our contention – a point we shall reiterate occasionally – that there is any organized male medical conspiracy against women patients. It is not as simple as that.

Chapter 3

Interpreting women's perceptions of menstruation

It should now be apparent that the medical perspective on menstruation and menstrual disorders is not only limited but also limiting. It is limited in the sense that the menstrual cycle has yet to yield many of its secrets to the biomedical sciences. It is limited also in relation to physicians' diagnostic and therapeutic decisions concerning disorders of the menstruum, many of which must be seen as conventional rather than rational. It is limiting in that the manner in which menstruation and menstrual disorders have been addressed in the biomedical sciences and clinical practice reflects the predominance of men amongst scientists and practitioners. The medical perspective remains essentially patriarchal.

In this chapter the focus is on women's ideas of normality and abnormality associated with menstruation, and especially on ways in which these diverge from those embedded in the medical perspective. Historical and anthropological studies are cited to illustrate continuities and discontinuities in women's beliefs and attitudes across time and cultures. Systematic attention is then paid to patterns of thinking about menstruation found in countries such as Britain and the USA, and to the difficulties of determining which circumstances cause women to regard themselves as suffering from menstrual symptoms.

CHANGING BELIEFS AND ATTITUDES

The term 'taboo' refers to prohibitions on behaviour which, if enacted, would threaten some or all of the relationships constituting the social world in which people live. It has been claimed that a *menstrual taboo* is common to almost all known epochs and cultures. Menstrual blood, in particular, has consistently been regarded as 'a volatile fluid capable of wide-ranging destruction' (Weideger 1975: 95). Hays (1972: 30) has shown how in many cultures women have been physically isolated during menstruation because of the perceived dangers of contact or contagion. He describes the convention of building special huts for women to occupy found among the Bakairi in Brazil, the Shusway in British Columbia, the Guari in Northern India, the Veddas in Ceylon and the Algonquin in North America, concluding that this convention 'covers the globe'.

The taboo may take other forms than isolation. In *The New Golden Bough* Frazer (1959: 212–13) recounts how in Uganda pots and pans handled or touched by a woman 'while the impurity of menstruation is upon her' have to be destroyed; and how among the Bribri Indians in Costa Rica a woman's food and drink are consumed from special containers carefully disposed of after use, 'for were a cow to find them, and eat them, it would waste away'. Elaborate rituals often have to be performed to purify an environment which has been defiled. Hays again:

> Among the Dogan of East Africa the menstrual taboo is so strong that a woman in this condition brings misfortune to everything she touches. Not only is she segregated in an isolated hut and provided with special eating utensils, but if she is seen passing through the village a general purification takes place.
>
> (1972: 30–1)

There is evidence also that in some cultures women have been punished for 'menstrual offences' prior to the carrying out of rituals of purification. In ancient Persia menstruation was judged to last four days, during which time a woman was isolated. If she was still menstruating after four days, she was given one hundred lashes and sent back into seclusion for a further five days. If she continued to menstruate after this second banishment, she received four hundred lashes because she was deemed to be 'possessed' by an evil spirit. Only then would purification rituals commence (Weideger 1975). In a few cultures – like that of the Illinois Indians – it is known that a woman could even forfeit her life for failing to give notice of menstruation (Novak 1921).

The ubiquity and potency of the menstrual taboo seems clear from historical and anthropological enquiries, but does it persist in modern industrial or post-industrial societies like Britain and the USA? There is evidence that it does. Snow and Johnson (1977) conducted a small pilot study of menstrual folklore among forty attenders at a clinic serving a multi-ethnic, low-income population in Ingham County, Michigan, USA. The women, many of them poorly educated, had little knowledge of the medical perspective on the menarche or the menstrual cycle: 62 per cent admitted to having no knowledge of menstruation prior to menarche; and 75 per cent lacked 'accurate information' about the onset of menses, 55

Table 3.1 Lack of understanding of the menstrual cycle

	Number of respondents	% of total sample
Do not know reason for menstruation	111	55.5
Do not know source of menstrual blood	67	33.5
Do not know when it is possible to become pregnant	127	63.5
Do not know 'safe time' for intercourse without pregnancy	158	79.0
Do not know if women can become pregnant before return of menses after giving birth	40	20.0
Do not know if women can become pregnant while breastfeeding infants	120	60.0
Do not know if pregnancy can occur during menopausal years	74	37.0
Avoid intercourse during menstruation	162	81.0

Source: Johnson and Snow 1982

per cent about the origin of menstrual flow, and 65 per cent about cessation of menstrual flow. A larger follow-up study, this time of 200 primarily low-income and poorly educated black women attending an inner-city antenatal clinic, again found considerable 'lack of understanding' of the menstrual cycle (see Table 3.1) (Johnson and Snow 1982).

Many of the women in Snow and Johnson's pilot investigation said they felt ashamed and embarrassed discussing menstruation with a physician. But if they were unfamiliar with the medical perspective and uncomfortable with physicians, there was no shortage of folklore interpretations of menstruation. One major theme of these was an association between menstruation and bodily cleanliness, 'the main purpose of the process being seen as to rid the system of impurities that might otherwise cause illness or poison the system' (1977: 2737). A number of women appeared to view the uterus as a hollow organ which is closed between menstrual episodes while it gradually fills with 'tainted blood'; it then opens up to permit the blood to escape during the menses. Some believed that women are most likely to become pregnant immediately before menstruation, when the uterus is beginning to open, during menstruation, when it is fully open, and immediately after menstruation, before it is tightly closed once more. At other times it seemed clear that the sperm would not be able to penetrate to allow conception to occur.

Sixty-two per cent of the sample believed that women should 'change their behaviour' during menstruation (or whenever vaginal bleeding is present). They prescribed caution. They felt that they were weak and vulnerable to illness at such times, largely because the opening of the uterus put them at risk from germs and other external entities (e.g. cold air or water). One young Mexican American woman believed that during menstruation 'the uterus is open, so you don't go to a funeral or you can catch cancer' (1977: 2738). She added that the germs of whatever the deceased died of might enter the open uterus to cause disease. Some black women became anxious during menstruation out of a belief that menstrual blood could be utilized to harm them through witchcraft.

Sixty-two per cent of women thought intercourse should be avoided during menstruation, not so much from a dislike of messiness or because they defined it as immoral, or even because they wanted to avoid pregnancy, but rather because it was seen as unhealthy, sometimes leading to increased flow, haemorrhage, infection and uterine cancer. Thirty-seven per cent believed that cold air and water should be avoided during menstruation because cold can arrest menstrual flow and result in life-threatening health problems: if normal flow does not occur, then the collected blood can enter the brain, causing insanity, a stroke or an oral haemorrhage (as in 'quick TB'). Interestingly, this view that obstructed menstrual flow renders women especially vulnerable and exposed to danger has been reported by Skultans (1970) in South Wales, where it was most common among women who thought menstrual bleeding good for their general health.

Twenty-two per cent of Snow and Johnson's sample favoured a change in diet during menstruation, notably the avoidance of cold foods like citrus fruits, tomatoes and green vegetables, again fearing impeded flow. Some other reactions to menstruation were reminiscent of the myths explicated by historians and anthropologists. Several Mexican American women, for example, expressed a fear of the *chirrionera* and the *ajolote*, lizard-like animals said to be attracted by the smell of menstrual blood and to attack menstruating women. 'Such a creature may forcibly enter the vagina and build a nest in the uterus; the hapless victim simulates pregnancy but gives birth to a litter of lizards or, in an alternate version, the animals eat the woman up on the inside and cause her to die' (1977: 2739). As many as 12 per cent of the total sample admitted to such fears.

What this study by Snow and Johnson indicates is that even in contemporary First-World societies women's beliefs and attitudes about menstruation may be profoundly negative, fearful and far removed from those of allopathic medicine. It might reasonably be argued, however, that the women in both their studies were from ethnic subcultures and poorly educated and therefore unrepresentative of women in the USA as a whole. We turn now to studies of women's interpretations of menstruation and menstrual disorders within what may be described as mainstream western culture.

CURRENT INTERPRETATIONS OF MENSTRUATION

Beliefs about menstruation tend to be acquired at an early age and 'usually reflect the general cultural stereotypes about menstruation as a negative and symptom-laden phenomenon' (Woods *et al*. 1982: 285). Clark and Ruble (1978) discovered that premenarcheal girls and boys of the same age associated numerous symptoms with the menstrual cycle. Whisnant and Zegans (1965) found that when white, middle-class adolescent girls in the USA were invited to describe their reactions to their first menstrual period, they typically used words like 'scared', 'upset' and 'ashamed'. Several studies of adult women's recollections of menarche confirm these negative feelings (e.g. Shainess 1961).

It is difficult to avoid the conclusions either that these negative beliefs and attitudes are a function of early cultural socialization or that the family is the principal agent of transmission (see chapter 5). Deutsch writes,

Menstruation is very often the one thing that the mother conceals from her children with particular discretion; it is a secret, and the idea of revealing it meets with great psychological resistance on her part. Many mothers find it much easier to talk with their daughters about conception, pregnancy, and birth than about menstruation.

(1944: 156)

Greer graphically recalls her own experience:

The arrival of menarche is more significant than any birthday, but in the Anglo-Saxon households it is ignored and carefully concealed from general awareness. For six months while I was waiting for my first menstruation I toted a paper bag with diapers and pins in my school satchel. When it finally came, I suffered agonies lest anyone should guess or *smell* it or anything. My diapers were made of harsh towelling, and I used to creep into the laundry and crouch over a bucket of foul clouts, hoping that my brother would not catch me at my revolting labours. It is not surprising that well-bred, dainty little girls find it difficult to adapt to menstruation, when our society does no more than explain it and leave them to get on with it.

(1971: 50)

Weideger (1975) also addresses the likely consequences for young girls:

> Adults consider it unpleasant, messy, and downright unclean. This assessment of menstruation is yet another nail in the coffin of female self-respect. The one salvation, the one source of equality her body provides is bound up with something corrupt and tainted. This is the lesson of menarche, and disappointment is the mildest of responses.

Woods and her colleagues (1982) found that adult women's recollections of menarche reflected a general ambivalence. Fifty-eight per cent reported being happy, 65 per cent proud, and 75 per cent excited. However, most women also recalled negative feelings: 67 per cent reported being upset, 82 per cent embarrassed, 29 per cent angry, and 74 per cent scared. Interestingly, 80 per cent also said they had been surprised at menarche. It has sometimes been claimed that negative feelings at the time – or negative recollections – of menarche may be associated with subsequent negative attitudes towards menstruation and symptom experience, although Woods and her co-workers found no evidence of this. They did find an association between current attitudes towards menstruation and current symptom experience, but they prudently counsel extreme caution in interpretating all data in this area.

Scambler and Scambler (1985) asked a sample of 79 women in London a number of questions relating to their attitudes towards menstruation. The women were encouraged to give expression to any positive or negative feelings they may have had. An analysis of their responses suggested three broad categories of attitude, which were termed 'acceptance', 'fatalism' and 'antipathy'.

Acceptance (25 per cent of women)

This category contained those women who reported experiencing no menstrual symptoms or who were only marginally affected by them. They saw their periods as essentially ' normal' occurrences:

> It's a normal, healthy thing; everybody has one.
>
> I just accept it as part of the process of life.
>
> I just don't take no notice of it really.

Those who did experience symptoms either thought nothing of them or played them down. This was the category where women came nearest to displaying a positive attitude towards menstruation, some referring to it as 'healthy' or 'feminine'. Even these women, however, often seemed to feel that their attitudes were exceptional or deviant, that what was generally expected of women was an altogether more negative assessment. Some clearly derived some satisfaction from their non-conformity, while others were almost apologetic that they had escaped the distress that everyone else seemed to experience.

Fatalism (27 per cent of women)

In this category were women who defined their periods as a 'nuisance', although they always qualified their statements:

> Well I wouldn't want to be without it . . . it's something you just live with, isn't it? They are a nuisance but I'd rather have them than not.

> I'm indifferent: I know I've got to have them so I put up with them.

> Well, I suppose it's a necessary evil so a woman can have a baby.

These women were resigned to menstruation. It was perceived as an essential part of being female, if not of being feminine.

Antipathy (48 per cent of women)

In this category were all those women who gave evidence of an unqualified or unconditional dislike of menstruation. This dislike ranged from negative feelings of inconvenience on the one hand, to strong feelings of disgust on the other. It was generally based on perceptions of menstruation as 'unhealthy', 'unclean', 'messy', and so on:

> I don't like them. I'd rather not have them. It's messy and I don't like mess. It's not a thing I enjoy talking about!

> I'd rather not have them at all . . . I just think it's messy: it doesn't seem fair to the woman.

> I don't like it. I suppose physically it doesn't affect me much, but mentally I don't like it at all.

> I don't bloody like them. I think it's because I have so much trouble with them – all the backaches and the stomach aches and the heavy bleeding. I've had so many problems with it ever since I started.

> I think it's a horrible mess!

Not surprisingly perhaps, a higher proportion of women showing antipathy towards menstruation were experiencing a high level of symptom distress (76 per cent) than was the case with women showing either fatalism (45 per cent) or acceptance (40 per cent). This is of course consistent with the finding reported by Wood and colleagues that current attitudes towards menstruation may be associated with current symptom experience (although no decisive statement can be made about the direction of causality).

Having briefly reviewed current attitudes, we now turn to women's experience of menstrual symptomatology, a field, as was implied in chapters 1 and 2, fraught with difficulty.

WOMEN'S EXPERIENCE OF MENSTRUAL SYMPTOMS

In the early 1960s, Kessel and Coppen bemoaned the fact that so little effort had been made to assess the prevalence of menstrual symptoms in the community. They rejected the view that women's own assessments of their symptoms were unreliable: 'Only the patient experiences her symptoms. Who else can be competent to assess them?' (1963: 61). Standardized questionnaires were completed by a sample of 465 women, focusing on pain, irritability, depression, anxiety, nervousness or tension, and headaches. The women were asked to rate these symptoms on a four-point scale: nil, slight, moderate, and severe. They were also asked about swelling of the body, whether it occurred and, if so, in what site. For each symptom they were asked the time in relation to menstruation when it was worst, and whether they suffered from it between periods.

Eighty-two per cent of the women had regular periods; 3 per cent were unsure whether they were regular or not; and 16 per cent were so irregular that they were unable to predict the next period. The prevalence of symptoms was as follows: 45 per cent reported moderate or severe pain; 22 per cent moderate or severe headache; 32 per cent moderate or severe irritability; and 23 per cent moderate or severe depression, anxiety, nervousness or tension. Seventy-two per cent said they experienced some swelling.

Kessel and Coppen found that certain symptoms – irritability, depression and tension, headache and body swelling – clustered 'in a temporal relationship': 'They are all maximal one or more days before the period begins, and they are significantly intercorrelated, so that a woman who experiences one is likely to experience the others' (1963: 63). The authors felt justified in following Frank and referring to a premenstrual syndrome (see chapter 1). Their figures suggested that the syndrome occurred to a moderate or severe degree in about a quarter of the women.

Pain was more common during than before menstruation, although their analysis led Kessel and Coppen to suggest that 'one type of period pain occurs premenstrually and can be regarded as an uncommon feature

Table 3.2 Menstrual symptoms most frequently defined as distressing

Before period		During period		Either before or during period or both	
Symptom	% Reporting as distressing	Symptom	% Reporting as distressing	Symptom	% Reporting as distressing
Irritability	38	Irritability	29	Irritability	49
Swelling	24	Pain	23	Pain	30
Headache	22	Fatigue	22	Fatigue	28
Depression	19	Depression	18	Moods	28
Moods	19	Moods	18	Swelling	27
Weight gain	19	Backache	15	Headache	25
Fatigue	18	Headache	14	Depression	24
Tension	15	Swelling	13	Weight gain	22
Backache	14	Weight gain	13	Backache	20
Tender breasts	14	Anxiety	11	Lowered performance	19
Pain	13	Avoidance of social activity	11	Tension	18
Anxiety	11	Lowered performance	11	Anxiety	16
				Avoidance of social activity	16

Source: Scambler and Scambler 1985

of the premenstrual syndrome, while the more usual type is worst during the period and is not part of the syndrome' (1963: 63).

This study indicated to many that menstrual symptoms were much more common than had been appreciated. It was followed by a sequence of surveys in the USA, Britain and elsewhere, many of the later ones deploying Moos's 47-item Menstrual Distress Questionnaire (MMDQ) (Moos 1968: 1977). Scambler and Scambler (1985) used a modified form of the MMDQ as one of several methodological tools in their study, reducing the original 47 items or symptoms to 34, according to a procedure adopted by Clare and Wiggins (1979). The women in their community sample were asked to rate each of the 34 symptoms for 'an average period' on a six-point scale: nil, barely noticeable, mild, moderate, strong, or acute. They did this for each phase of the menstrual cycle: the premenstruum, the menstruum, and the remainder of the cycle. Any symptom defined as strong or acute was regarded as distressing.

Table 3.2 gives the rank order of the symptoms most frequently defined as distressing during the seven days preceding menstruation, during the menstrual flow, and during either or both of these phases. While no attempt was made to test Kessel and Coppen's notion of a premenstrual syndrome, it can be seen that the findings here are broadly consonant with those of the earlier survey in terms of the distributions of symptoms over the premenstrual and menstrual phases. In all, 82 per cent of the women in Scambler and Scambler's study rated at least one symptom as distressing; 15 per cent suffered distress in the premenstruum only, 9 per cent during the flow only, and 58 per cent during both phases.

An overall menstrual distress score was also calculated. A woman scored one point for each of the 34 symptoms she defined as strong or acute during the seven days prior to menstruation. When totalled, these gave her a premenstrual distress score. The same procedure was followed for symptoms defined as strong or acute during the menstrual flow. When totalled, these gave her a menstrual flow distress score. A combined or overall menstrual distress score was achieved by adding these two scores together. This meant that a woman who experienced distress from an individual symptom both before and during the menstrual flow had her overall menstrual distress score automatically weighted to allow for distress over time as well as for its intensity. Any woman with an overall menstrual distress score of four or more was said to have a 'high' level of symptom distress. Fifty-four per cent came into this category. As many as 28 per cent had an overall menstrual distress score of eight or more. As expected, women using oral contraceptives were less likely to experience a high level of symptom distress (38 per cent) than were other members of the sample (60 per cent).

Although these findings are fairly representative of other similar work, there are a number of problems concerning their interpretation that need to be acknowledged. Three of the many studies conducted in the 1970s and 1980s have been picked out for discussion here, because together they clearly demonstrate the dangers of accepting at face value the findings from all studies utilizing questionnaires which incorporate and require responses to check-lists of menstrual symptoms.

The first study was conducted by Parlee and was designed to consider the 'methodological soundness' of the Moos MDQ. Parlee gave small samples of women and men the MMDQ 'with instructions to indicate what women experience during the menstrual cycle' (1974: 239). She found that women and men gave very similar reports of the kinds of 'symptom changes' occurring before and during menstruation. Moreover, the reports of the women and men in Parlee's study were comparable to those of the women in a study by Moos. Moos (1969) unambiguously interpreted the reports of the women in his study as indicating 'complaints' of 'symptoms'. Parlee conveys this process of interpretation as follows:

> Differences between reports of individuals were interpreted as evidence that 'different women have tendencies to get symptoms in different areas' (Moos 1969: 400) and that 'some women appear to have dysmenorrhea (high menstrual pain scores) but no premenstrual tension, whereas others have premenstrual tension (high premenstrual negative affect) but no menstrual pain, and still others have both dysmenorrhea and premenstrual tension' (ibid.).

It may be, Parlee admits, that the reports of the women in her study should be interpreted in this same way. But how would one then account for the reports of the men? Perhaps the women were reporting their direct personal experiences ('albeit projected outward to apply to *women*') while the men were reporting the symptoms which they had 'learned' through 'a myriad of social sources' to associate with menstruation. But would this explain the 'very high correlations' between the male and female reports? Parlee thinks it 'extremely unlikely' and puts forward an alternative hypothesis. She suggests that questionnaires like the MMDQ provide measures of 'stereotypic conceptions of menstrual distress or premenstrual tension' (1974: 239). In other words, the MMDQ merely taps a pervasive cultural stereotype of menstrual symptomatology.

The second study to be described was undertaken by AuBuchon and Calhoun (1985), largely to examine the effects of 'social expectancy' on the reporting of menstrual cycle symptomatology. A small sample of healthy women with regular cycles were randomly assigned to two groups, one of which was told that menstrual symptoms were the focus of the study, and the other of which was not. A control group of men was also included. All participants in the study were tested twice weekly for eight weeks on a check-list of symptoms. The results indicated that those women who had been told that it was a study of menstrual symptoms reported significantly more negative psychological and somatic symptoms at the premenstrual and menstrual phases than did the other two groups. In fact, those women not told the nature of the study reported a very similar pattern of symptoms to that reported by the men. AuBuchon and Calhoun conclude that social expectancy has a considerable effect on the reporting of menstrual symptoms.

The final study also focused on social expectancies, but differed from the second in that an attempt was made both to manipulate women's expectancies for a 'negative mood–menstrual relationship' and to assess the impact of these manipulated expectancies on moods reported daily during the course of one complete menstrual cycle (Olasov and Jackson 1987). The college women recruited to the study were randomly assigned to one of four groups: the first viewed a videotaped lecture designed to increase expectancies for a negative mood–menstrual relationship; the second viewed a lecture designed to decrease such expectancies; the third were exposed to a lecture on an unrelated topic; and the fourth, a blind control group, was neither exposed to a lecture nor aware that the study was concerned with the menstrual cycle. Expectancies were assessed immediately before and after the presentation of the lectures. In addition, the women in all four groups monitored their moods for forty consecutive days, after which expectancies were once again assessed.

Olasov and Jackson predicted that the impact of the manipulations on expectancies would be evident both immediately and at the forty day follow-up assessment. More specifically, they hypothesized that the (first) group manipulated so as to increase expectancies for a negative mood–menstrual relationship would both report the most negative moods during the forty days of self-monitoring, and report expectancies for the most negative moods at the forty day follow-up assessment. And they hypothesized that the second group, manipulated so as to decrease expectancies for a negative mood–menstrual relationship, would both report the most positive moods during the forty days of self-monitoring, and report expectancies for the most positive moods at the forty day follow-up assessment. The remaining, third and fourth, groups, it was hypothesized, would be intermediate between these two. These hypotheses were corroborated. In other words, it seems clear first, that expectancies can be altered by means of a brief lecture (the effects remaining discernible over a period of at least forty days); and second, that altered expectancies affect the reporting of daily moods throughout the menstrual cycle.

There can be little doubt then that reports of menstrual symptomatology, especially when obtained through instruments like the MMDQ, reflect and bring to the surface women's – often stereotypical and negative – attitudes and expectancies relating to menstruation. As part of Scambler and Scambler's (1985) study women were asked to keep a six-week health diary and to record daily any changes in health status; they were not told beforehand of any particular interest in menstruation. Only 58 per cent of the women made any reference to their periods in the diaries, while it will be recalled that 82 per cent of the same women subsequently rated at least one symptom as severe on the MMDQ. As we have seen, it may also be the case that women's expectancies can be modified by planned interventions.

In the final section of this chapter we reflect further on the nature of the links between women's lay and men's medical perspectives on menstruation and menstrual problems, and suggest some analytic distinctions which may have heuristic value.

ALTERED STATES, ILLNESS AND DISEASE

According to the medical perspective, physicians' interest in menstruation is largely confined to screening for, diagnosing and, if appropriate, treating disease. In pursuit of such ends they rely very substantially on women's presentations of menstrual complaints or symptoms. Although much of what physicians think and do is not explicable in terms of the medical perspective (see chapter 4), it is reasonable to characterize their approach as disease-oriented and as hinging predominantly on symptoms presented in their surgeries or clinics.

The word 'illness' is conventionally used in place of disease to denote lay, in this case women's, conceptualizations of health-related problems. Whilst lay conceptualizations of illness may on occasions correspond precisely to medical conceptualizations of disease, this need not be the case. Indeed, there will be many times when women see themselves as suffering symptoms of menstrual illness in the absence of menstrual disease; and other times when women do not perceive themselves to be experiencing symptoms of illness despite the presence of menstrual disease.

It should be acknowledged immediately that, for all its usefulness, this distinction between disease and illness can represent an oversimplification of complex phenomena. Higgins (1984: 728) has shown this from a clinician's viewpoint in his examination of 'those individuals who present to doctors with symptoms suggesting physical disease but in whom no physical disease can be found or in whom physical disease, if present, does not fully explain their symptoms: what might be called mimicked disease or pseudo-disease'. He adds, 'Hidden in the camouflage of disease, these patients are not what they seem.' The kinds of issues raised by Higgins follow on from much of the discussion in this chapter and will be taken up directly in chapter 4.

It is apparent, however, that many women do not understand the changes occurring with menstruation as forms of illness. Instead of symptoms of illness they discern indications of *altered states*. Indeed, as suggested earlier, some positively welcome menstruation. Weideger (1975: 4–5) cites the following comments:

> It [menstruation] makes me very much aware of the fact that I am a woman, and that's something very important to me. . . . It's also a link to other women. I actually enjoy having my period. I feel like I've been cleaned out inside.
>
> The menstrual cycle has become such a part of my life by now, I don't want to change it. It is part of being a woman, which I am proud to be.
>
> I really like it. It's difficult to explain, but it's the same way I like the changing of the seasons. I guess the monthly cycles are 'earthy' and symbolic to me.

Even unwelcome menstrual change may be interpreted in terms of indications of altered states rather than symptoms of illness. Inconvenience and discomfort, although negatively evaluated, need not be linked with failures of health.

Figure 3.1 sets out a provisional analytic framework within which women's perceptions of menstrual change might be accommodated. It should be emphasized once more that it is seen as of heuristic value. Women's perceptions might often be mixed, and need not remain constant over time.

If these distinctions have any usefulness, this should be apparent in any consideration of women's health, illness and consulting behaviour in relation to menstruation; and it is to such issues that we now turn.

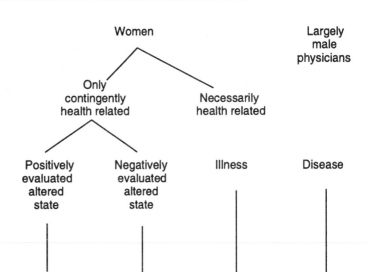

Figure 3.1 An analytic framework for women's perceptions of menstrual change

Chapter 4

Women and help-seeking

This chapter is concerned with what women do in response to menstrual change, especially when such change is interpreted in terms of symptoms of illness. The early sections have to do with the circumstances in which women typically appraise change. Attention is paid to their use of social networks and to the likely impact of the networks on decision-making. Kleinman's (1985) model of 'local health care systems' is cited to show that consulting a physician is only one of several options open to women experiencing menstrual discomfort.

Also discussed are physician consultation rates for problems perceived to be associated with menstruation, and women's experiences and judgements of medical consultations.

APPRAISING CHANGE

The principal focus of this chapter is on 'illness behaviour', that is, on the circumstances in which women define menstrual change in terms of symptoms of illness, and what, if anything, they do in consequence. The difficulties of interpreting women's reports of menstrual symptoms have already been noted. In particular, we have seen that reports obtained through the MMDQ may reflect women's learned negative stereotypes and attitudes to menstruation as much as their experiences of it. Hence the finding in Scambler and Scambler's (1985) study that fewer than three out of five women, when unaware of the researchers' interest in menstruation, recorded their periods in six-week health diaries, while more than four out of five of the same women rated at least one menstrual symptom as distressing when confronted by the MMDQ.

When Scambler and Scambler invited women in their sample to complete health diaries, they requested daily information on any disturbance of health; any conversations held with lay persons about their health; and any action taken as a consequence of any disturbance of health. No mention was made of menstruation until after the diaries had been collected. On collection, however, the women were interviewed in detail about their diary entries, and especially about those relating to menstruation. The material concerning menstrual attitudes was outlined in the previous chapter. But the women were also probed on their perceptions of menstrual change as illness and on the effects of menstrual change on quality of life.

Menstrual change as illness

Fifty-eight per cent of the women recorded their periods in their health diaries, and this was taken as prima-facie evidence of a perceived association with illness. When questioned, several volunteered comments such as:

It's a special female illness; I don't think it's normal.

It has to happen to women, but I'd code it as an illness.

It's an illness that only happens to women. It's something that comes over you, and, to me, if something comes over you, that's an illness.

It's a female illness: that's how it makes you feel.

Three themes are apparent in remarks like these: first, menstruation was seen by these women as constituting a readily discernible – bodily – change; second, this change 'felt like', or was at least analagous to, an episode of illness; and third, there was a clear link in their outlook between the perception of menstruation as illness and an attitude of 'antipathy' towards it (see chapter 3).

Many of those who did not mention their periods in their diaries were surprised to be probed on their exclusion:

You said anything healthwise: I didn't consider *that* something to do with my health!

I don't class it as an illness – not as unwell – so I didn't put it down.

Other more general comments suggested either that menstruation was normal but a nuisance:

I don't think it's a sickness or illness. I think of it as inconvenient but *normal*.

I would say it's normal – normal and healthy, but inconvenient.

> It's normal really, isn't it? It does you good. . . . Oh, it's a nuisance. I don't feel, sort of, free when I have a period: I can't come and go as I like. It's like having a load of rules – you can't do this and you can't do that!

or that it was normal and non-intrusive:

> You see, it doesn't bother *me*, so I don't really bother about *it*.

> It's perfectly normal: I don't even think about them.

> I'd be more concerned if I didn't [i.e. menstruate]. . . . When I missed one period on the pill I wasn't happy then. You know you've got to flush out once a month; I have that feeling anyway.

Women who regarded menstruation as normal, rejecting any association with illness, typically displayed attitudes of either 'fatalism', if they saw it as a nuisance, or 'acceptance', if they saw it as non-intrusive (see chapter 3).

Menstrual change and quality of life

The women were also questioned about the extent to which menstruation had an impact on the quality of their lives. Forty-three per cent said that it definitely diminished quality of life. The remainder reported either that it had no impact on quality of life at all (19 per cent):

> I don't think they affect me at all.

> No, all it does is tell me I'm going through a certain stage.

or – twice as many – that any such impact was negligible (38 per cent):

> It doesn't affect my life, but it can be a nuisance; I suppose all women must think that.

All of the women who stated unambiguously that the quality of their lives was negatively affected specified the principal areas of life that were disrupted. These fell into four categories: 41 per cent (18 per cent of the total sample) said that it adversely affected their *mental state*; 38 per cent (16 per cent of the total sample) specified their *social life*; 15 per cent (6 per cent of the total sample) specified their *sex life*; and 6 per cent (3 per cent of the total sample) specified their *physical state* (e.g. pain). Examples of statements include:

> Yes, I'm waiting for that week to come when I know I'm going to feel terrible. I dread it, I *really* dread it. I'm hateful: I upset the whole family.

It does for a few days: I get very tired and don't want to go out.

I don't want to go out, even when going to work, because I can't get clothes on!

I don't like having them because I like to go swimming. . . . I feel as though it's showing, you know, it's really funny, and I sort of stand in the corner and don't move.

It affects your moods and therefore your life.

Yes, I think so, especially – like it can affect the marriage and things like that, like at that particular time of the month they don't want you.

I never have sex when I'm like that.

There was a strong association between putative definitions of menstruation as illness and judgements that it diminished quality of life. Eighty-one per cent of those who appeared from their diary entries to relate menstruation to illness said that their periods negatively affected the quality of their lives, compared with only 19 per cent of those who omitted to mention menstruation in their diaries. Interestingly also, there were statistically significant associations between a high level of symptom distress on the shortened version of the MMDQ (see chapter 3) and both perceptions of menstruation as illness and judgements of diminished quality of life (Scambler 1980).

The findings of this and other studies, several of them reviewed earlier, are consistent with the following theoretical statement about women's accounts of menstrual change, although they by no means confirm it. Against the background of the menstrual taboo, which remains salient – if in muted form – in patriarchal societies such as Britain and the USA, early family socialization induces young girls to anticipate and experience menarche with apprehension. It is through their silence about menarche and menstruation that parents in particular may function as 'stigma coaches', signalling secrecy and shame (Schneider and Conrad 1980: 36). A momentous social transition is often simply ignored. Menarche is a *rite de passage* largely without celebration.

Trained through neglect to perceive menstruation as something unpleasant, undesirable and to be concealed, many women are primed to reflect and reproduce cultural stereotypes by associating it with distress – often with symptoms of illness – and to view it as disruptive of the quality of their lives. The experience of unpredictable menstrual change or of psychological or somatic discomfort may consolidate this perspective; the experience of predictable, benign menstrual change or of some form of re-socialization may undermine it. The relationship between menstrual attitudes and menstrual experience is almost certainly an interactive one (i.e. each influences the other in an ongoing dialectical fashion).

LAY REFERRAL AND LOCAL HEALTH CARE SYSTEMS

There is a tendency in the medical literature and outside it to assume that people's definitions of illness echo physicians' definitions of disease, and that when people come to regard themselves as ill they are predisposed to seek physicians' help. The reality is more complex. Not only can there be radical disjunctions between lay and professional thinking on health-related problems and issues, but people who define themselves as ill rarely anticipate, let alone secure, consultations with physicians. Nor are consultations merely a function of the severity of symptoms. While studies do indeed suggest that the greater the symptom severity the more likely it is that consultations with physicians will occur (e.g. Ingham and Miller 1979), there is no doubt either that many severe symptoms do not precipitate consultations or that significant numbers of treatable diseases are unseen by physicians (hence Last's (1963) coining of the term 'clinical iceberg', referring to the fact that physicians only see the tip of the iceberg of disease).

Emphasizing the fact that people have and deploy options other than consulting physicians, Kleinman introduces the notion of the multi-dimensional 'local health care system'. Figure 4.1 displays the three main arenas of care that constitute a local health care system: *popular, folk* and *professional*. As the figure implies, most symptoms of illness are accommodated within the popular (or lay) health care sector.

Kleinman writes of the popular arena: 'here *illness* is first experienced, labelled, and treated by the individual (self-care), or more often by family members and other members of the social network' (1985: 142). The popular sector subsumes a wide variety of practices, including health maintenance and curative interventions,

> of which the most commonly utilized are diet; special foods; local herbs and other traditional and contemporary indigenous medicines; massage; blistering and other manipulative techniques; exercise; changes in life style habits; use of biomedical drugs and apparatuses; symbolic interventions, ranging from charms and amulets to prayer, healing rites, and including various kinds of talking therapies.
>
> (1985: 142)

Little is known about the extent of the use (or the effects) of such healing practices in relation to menstrual symptoms, although Westcott (1987)

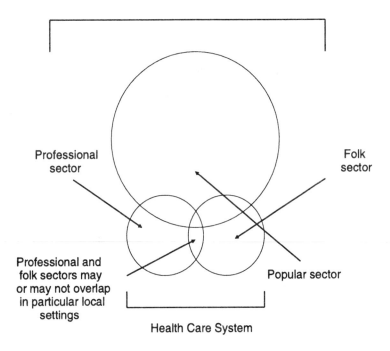

Figure 4.1 Local health care system
Source: Kleinman 1985

has listed several 'alternative' treatments for medically-defined menstrual disorders. These treatments tend to be available and in use in the popular sector, but some are typically administered from the folk sector, that is, by non-professional, non-bureaucratized 'specialists'. Like many folk practitioners, Westcott argues that women should generally seek clearance or advice from physicians before embarking upon the more esoteric of the alternative remedies.

Westcott discusses amenorrhoea, menorrhagia, dysmenorrhoea and premenstrual syndrome. Alternative therapies for amenorrhoea include homoeopathy and acupuncture. Herbal treatment, usually accessible through folk practitioners, is also available. Garden sage (*salvia officinalis*) is used for regulating periods; and chaste tree or monk's pepper (*vitex agnus castus*) is used when appropriate to achieve hormonal rebalance. Changes in diet are often recommended for menorrhagia in the belief that a lack of vitamin A can be a causal factor. Iron-rich foods such as green vegetables, wheat-germ, liver and parsley are used to counteract possible anaemia due to excessive blood loss. Both acupuncture and osteopathy are employed, as again are herbal remedies.

Common forms of self-help for dysmenorrhoea include holding a covered hot water bottle against the abdomen; taking a warm bath or shower; relaxation techniques; exercise, especially swimming, dancing or yoga; and the direct massage of the uterus (i.e. by pressing into the abdomen just above the pubic hairs and massaging gently). Herbal treatments such as raspberry leaf tea can be used. Homoeopathic remedies embrace calc carb (for sore breasts), calc phos (for headache), lycopodium (for depression), nat mur (for irritability) and pulsatilla (for weepiness and painful breasts). Other interventions listed by Westcott include acupuncture, osteopathy, acupressure, Shiatsu massage, aromatherapy and nutritional remedies.

Westcott contends that the boundaries between medical and alternative treatments are more blurred in the case of premenstrual syndrome than for amenorrhoea, menorrhagia and dysmenorrhoea. This is true of diet for example, which has engaged medical researchers and clinicians as well as folk practitioners. Herbal remedies may be apposite, as may homoeopathic treatments: to the list cited under dysmenorrhoea can be added graphites (for weight gain) and sepia (for mood swings). Acupuncture and acupressure are used. Headaches may be combated through reducing alcohol intake; cutting out certain types of food (e.g. cheese and dairy products); and taking regular meals.

As Kleinman points out, the popular sector of care is also

> where help-seeking decisions are made in the lay referral network regarding when to go to a particular practitioner for care, which practitioner to visit, whether to change practitioners or seek therapeutic alternatives, how long to remain in treatment, whether or not to comply with therapeutic recommendations, and how to assess outcome.
>
> (1985: 142)

We shall concentrate here on the role of lay referral networks in either prompting women with perceived menstrual problems to enter the professional arena of a local health care system (i.e. consult a physician) or inhibiting them from doing so.

It was Freidson (1970) who first argued that help-seeking decisions are organized by lay referral networks or systems. It is clearly routine for people who define themselves as ill to consult other lay persons, to discuss symptoms or to seek advice (Scambler and Scambler 1984). In one study in the USA, Suchman (1965) found that three-quarters of the

Table 4.1 Lay consultants for general and menstrual symptoms

Type of lay consultants	General symptoms (% of lay consultations)	Menstrual symptoms (% of lay consultations)
Husband	50	58
Mother	10	16
Other female kin	8	8
Female friends	25	12
Other	7	6
Total	100	100

symptoms presented to physicians had first been discussed with lay persons, usually relatives. Scambler and her colleagues (1981) report the same finding; and they add that over the six weeks that the women in their study maintained health diaries, an average of eleven lay consultations were registered for every one medical consultation (a ratio which almost certainly understates the frequency of lay consulting).

Scambler and her associates found that all the women in their sample recorded lay consultations in their health diaries. Half the women recorded lay consultations for menstrual symptoms. Table 4.1 gives breakdowns of types of lay consultant for both general and menstrual symptoms. It can be seen that the breakdowns are very similar. Perhaps the most conspicuous difference is that proportionately more lay consultations for menstrual symptoms (80 per cent) than for general symptoms (68 per cent) took place within the family. A related, and perhaps surprising, finding is that fewer lay consultations for menstrual symptoms (12 per cent) than for general symptoms (25 per cent) were with female friends.

The interviews conducted on the completion of the health diaries elicited three main types of lay consultations about menstrual symptoms: *casual*, *enquiring* and *confirmatory*. Casual consultations were nothing more than items buried in everyday conversation, unplanned and largely without significance for future action. Many consultations with husbands were of this type. Enquiring consultations were quests for information or advice, frequently tapping the known experience of others; these were almost exclusively with other women, like mothers, sisters or friends. Confirmatory consultations amounted to requests for support, often in relation to decisions already made; thus one woman explained,

> I probably told her so that I would make sure of going to the doctor ...
> you know, because I was in two minds whether to go or not, and she

said, 'Oh go. You must go to the doctor.' And I think that's probably why I told her.

This woman's confirmatory consultation may be interpreted as an expressed need for what Zola (1973) has called 'sanctioning', that is, pressure from others to consult a physician.

The research literature does not permit clear statements about links between lay referral networks and lay consultations and help-seeking behaviour for menstrual symptoms in either the folk or the professional sectors of local health care systems. Scambler and Scambler were able to show, however, that at least one property of women's networks did appear to influence whether or not they made appointments to enter the professional sector. Networks were analysed in numerous different ways, for example in terms of their size, composition and proximity to women's homes. The most convincing link with general practitioner consultations for menstrual symptoms involved women's active kinship networks.

Women with large active kinship networks – that is, women with four or more kin whom they met or spoke to on the telephone at least once a week – were significantly more likely to have consulted their general practitioners for menstrual symptoms during the year prior to interview than women with small active kinship networks. This mirrors the finding for general, as opposed to merely menstrual, symptoms. It may be, then, that women who enjoy a high rate of contact with kin routinely have highly focused, and sometimes protracted, discussions about menstrual and other symptoms with them; and that – whether or not they seek it through confirmatory consultations – sanctioning is a common product of such dialogues. In other words, kin consultations about menstrual and other symptoms tend to lead to kin referrals to general practitioners and produce higher rates of use (Scambler *et al.* 1981: 749).

HELP-SEEKING AND THE PROFESSIONAL SECTOR

The point was made in chapter 1 that menstrual disorders rank amongst the ten conditions most frequently seen in general practice. In their community study, Scambler and Scambler (1985) found that 74 per cent of their sample of 79 women had at some time or other consulted their general practitioners for menstrual problems. Four per cent had consulted within a week before interview, 12 per cent within a month, 23 per cent within three months, 28 per cent within six months, 37 per cent within a year, 51 per cent within two years, 59 per cent within five years, and 74 per cent at some time since menarche; 26 per cent had never consulted any physician for menstrual difficulties.

The authors were particularly interested in factors associated with consulting general practitioners within the year before interview; they referred to the 37 per cent of women involved as *recent consulters*. None of the socio-demographic factors examined – for example, age, employment status, social class – were significantly associated with recent consulting. It has already been noted that large active kinship networks seemed to predispose to consulting. Interestingly, although a high level of symptom distress 'for an average period' (as measured by the shortened version of the Moos MDQ), a perceived negative effect on quality of life, and a perception of menstruation as illness, showed some association with recent consulting, none achieved association at a level of statistical significance (Scambler 1980).

These findings, and particularly the fact that over a half of women with a high level of symptom distress had not taken advantage of the professional sector of their local health care system for over a year, encouraged Scambler and Scambler (1985) to focus on 'non-consulters'. The 63 per cent who had not consulted within the year before interview seemed to fall into four main categories: the 'unaffected', the 'alienated', the 'realists' and the 'marginals'.

The unaffected (35 per cent of non-consulters)

This group of women neither associated menstruation with illness nor experienced symptoms or distress. None felt that their periods had adversely affected the quality of their lives. Most displayed attitudes of acceptance, although a few were fatalists.

It may be that these women would be unlikely or reluctant help-seekers in the event of any future distress, that they would tend to interpret distress as indicative of an altered state, sometimes a negatively evaluated one, rather than as symptomatic of illness.

The alienated (33 per cent of non-consulters)

This group associated menstruation with illness and experienced a high level of symptom distress. Almost all felt the quality of their lives had been affected, and most held antipathetic attitudes towards menstruation. Eighty per cent had presented menstrual symptoms to a physician in the past (i.e. more than a year before interview). Interestingly, working-class women were overrepresented in this group; indeed, 77 per cent were from families in which the principal earner was in semi-skilled or unskilled manual work, compared with 29 per cent of the total sample. It was a common perception amongst these women that medicine could afford them little or no relief from their symptom distress. Some judged they had been 'let down' by physicians in the past. Several had long-term symptoms which they had simply learned to 'put up with':

> I don't consult – I haven't bothered again – I don't feel they understand the problem and it's so hard to explain.

The realists (17 per cent of non-consulters)

This group linked menstruation with illness, but experienced little symptom distress. They did not regard their periods as having a negative impact on the quality of their lives, but tended to be fatalists rather than acceptors in attitude. It is probably reasonable to suggest that these women would be predisposed to seek professional help in the event of future distress.

The marginals (15 per cent of non-consulters)

This group did not think of menstruation as illness, but experienced high levels of symptom distress (although not as high as the alienated). They were almost equally split between those who accepted their periods and felt the quality of their lives to have been unaffected, and those who were antipathetic and judged the quality of their lives to have suffered. Less than half had had a menstrual consultation in the past, and these averaged more than five years before interview. Women from middle-class families were overrepresented in this group: 43 per cent belonged to families in which the principal earner was engaged in professional or managerial work, compared with 13 per cent of the total sample. Almost all the women expressed one or more of the following attitudes: a dislike of medicine, doctors and examinations; a preference for women doctors; and dissatisfaction with doctors in the past.

WOMEN AND THEIR PHYSICIANS

In a study of self-referral, Hannay (1980) found that 26 per cent of a random sample of people with symptoms which they defined as severely painful, disabling or serious did not consult a physician; conversely, 11 per cent of those with symptoms which they did not define as painful, disabling or serious did consult. He refers to 'incongruous' referral behaviour. From the preceding discussion it is clear that one cause of incongruous referral behaviour in relation to menstrual symptoms – in particular, not consulting despite high levels of menstrual distress – is unease or dissatisfaction with male physicians, or even with female physicians initiated and socialized into the predominantly male subculture of medicine. (See Young (1981): 'a woman doctor, whatever her job, is seen in our culture as an honorary man, simply by virtue of society's concept of what a doctor is'; and also chapter 2).

Several participants in Scambler and Scambler's study volunteered remarks such as:

> I'd possibly find it difficult. I don't think he'd [i.e. her GP] quite understand the same as a woman. That's how I feel: I'd find it easier to talk to a woman.

> If I haven't got to be examined I don't mind going to a man; but I feel that if I'm going to be examined I'd rather go to a woman.

> I wondered if I should go back and see a woman about it [i.e. premenstrual syndrome]. They've been through it; they may be in the same situation.

But not all women preferred female physicians for menstrual consultations. Indeed, one woman took exception to female physicians in precisely this context:

> I think women are not as understanding as men if you're not well. I can speak to a man probably better, but I think women doctors are inclined to think, 'Oh, I have the same problem, and if I've got to put up with it . . .'

In their survey of general practice, Cartwright and Anderson (1981) found that most people expressed no preference between male and female physicians for general symptoms. But when there was a preference, 20 per cent of the women preferred a female physician, and 25 per cent of men a male one; 3 per cent of women expressed a preference for a male physician. In Scambler and Scambler's study, 53 per cent of the women interviewed expressed no preference between male and female physicians when consulting for menstrual symptoms, 34 per cent preferred a female physician, and 13 per cent preferred a male physician. Preference was not related either to the gender of women's general practitioners or to whether or not they had consulted with menstrual symptoms in the year before the study. Circumstantial evidence from a variety of other studies suggests that women are more likely to prefer a female physician when presenting 'women's complaints' than at other times (Roberts 1985).

Scambler and Scambler also asked women how easy they would find it to talk to their general practitioners about menstrual problems. Just under half, 49 per cent, replied that it would be very easy, that it was not a problem; 28 per cent said that it would be 'quite easy', but implied that they would have some qualms; 19 per cent stated that they would find it rather difficult; and 4 per cent said that it would be 'very difficult'. None suggested that they would find it an impossible task. Once again, women's responses were unrelated either to the gender of their general practitioners or to whether or not they had consulted with menstrual symptoms in the year before the study (Scambler 1980).

The picture is a complicated one. Criticisms of male physicians – as well as of the institution of medicine itself – from women consulting for menstrual problems appear to be quite common. A third of women would prefer to see a female physician. A half of women would have reservations about discussing menstrual symptoms with their general practitioners, with nearly a quarter reporting that it would be either difficult or very difficult. However, we know of no systematic studies of physician–patient interaction during encounters featuring menstrual symptoms.

A few more analytic distinctions might be helpful at this juncture. Women such as the alienated identified above – namely, those who decline to enter, or re-enter, the professional sector despite associating menstruation with illness and experiencing a high level of symptom distress – appear to be motivated by one or more of three perceptions. The first is that physicians *lack empathy* with women who present with menstrual symptoms. This is partly explicable in terms of the formers' preoccupation with a largely biomedical conception of disease, but also relevant is the fact that both textbook and applied medicine remain discernibly sexist (see chapter 2).

The second perception is that physicians are *ignorant* of the menstrual cycle and of problems associated with it. Regardless of whether or not they appreciate or take seriously the complaints that women present with, their understanding of the processes of menstruation – generally obtained through biomedicine – is partial and often provisional. The third perception is related to the second, and is that physicians are *ineffective*. Whether through lack of empathy or ignorance or both, they are rarely able to offer rational therapies to end or ease menstrual distress.

If they are not to mislead, it is important that these three types or categories of perceptions are given some elaboration. First, they may be either *experiential* or *inferential*. They may be said to be experiential if they derive and are formed from experience, that is, if they are rooted in encounters with physicians who lacked empathy or were ignorant or ineffective. They may be described as inferential if they do not have their genesis in experience, but are inferences either from the experiences of others (i.e. members of women's lay referral networks or systems) or from related experiences of, for example, men or of male (or honorary male) physicians.

And second, they may be either *personal* or *generalized*. They can be characterized as personal if they apply only to particular physicians, like women's own general practitioners. They are more appropriately described as generalized if they are applied to all physicians, and hence to the institution of medicine itself. While there are probable empirical links between perceptions which are experiential and personal on the one hand, and between perceptions which are inferential and generalized on the other, these are not of course logical – or necessary – links. It is clearly possible, for example, for women's perceptions to be experiential (i.e. derived from experience) and generalized (i.e. extended to all physicians and to medicine).

The urgent need remains for substantive research to test the value of analytic distinctions like these. But it is now time to consider in more detail the accommodation of menstrual change in the context of personal and social relationships, especially with men and in nuclear family units (chapter 5); and in the context of social, educational and employment activities outside the home (chapter 6).

Chapter 5

Menstrual change and relationships with men

It seems clear that many girls are coached by their mothers, who may be unaware of the salience and pervasiveness of patriarchal ideology, to see menarche and menstrual change not as celebrations of their maturity and womanhood, but as embarrassing intrusions into their lives, as phenomena best acknowledged and accommodated in private with a minimum of fuss. They are phenomena, moreover, which neither boys nor men can be expected to know about or comprehend; they belong in the female domain. This chapter analyses the extent to which such perceptions survive into marriages of procreation and the impact of both perception and menstrual change and disorder on family relationships, especially between spouses. Special attention is given to the premenstrual syndrome – or premenstrual tension (PMT) as it is more commonly known – and to sexuality and menstruation. A discussion of recent research on attitudes to menstruation in male culture is incorporated.

WOMEN'S UNDERSTANDING OF PMT

The following statement about premenstrual irritability by one of the women interviewed by Scambler and Scambler is paradigmatic in a number of respects:

> Sometimes I come home and snap, and he says, 'Oh yes, your period's due next week.' He's thought about it before I have. His reactions don't help. I've got no control over it. I know I'm doing it as well: I can stand outside myself and watch myself doing it.

First, because of its timing, the putative change of mood is linked with menstruation and thence interpreted either as an indication of a negatively evaluated altered state or as a symptom of illness (see chapter 3). Second, it is the behaviour of a man – typically, as in this case, the husband –

which is crucial, even decisive, in both identifying and interpreting a change of mood. And third, these processes of identification and interpretation are telling largely due to the 'medicalization' of premenstrual change as premenstrual syndrome.

What precisely is implied in this analysis? The ground was prepared in chapter 2. It is certainly not being denied that many women may experience change in the form of discomfort or distress in the few days prior to the menstruum. However, as has been argued, some may well be predisposed through socialization to associate, or to accept others associating, negative feelings – like irritability – rather than positive feelings with their periods. Taylor makes the point that no research teams have 'systematically described or studied the positive effects of menstruation' (1988: 58). And she adds of the Moos Menstrual Distress Questionnaire, 'If a woman did feel positively about any part of her period, there would be no place to put it on this questionnaire.' In one of the very few forays into the general area of positively evaluated altered states, Hopson and Rosenfeld (1984) have in fact estimated that 12 per cent of women experience positive change during menstruation, including increased energy, sensitivity and creativity, heightened arousal and desire for sex, and a general feeling of well-being.

As the following quotations from Weideger's (1975: 49–50) respondents in the USA suggest, a wide range of predominantly negative states and symptoms are typically identified in studies of menstruating women:

Approximately one week prior, I bloat up, feel fat and klutzy, get very irritable, cramps, back and leg aches during.

No real distress except melancholy which I actually enjoy. It's a quiet reflective time for me.

My skin breaks out around both ovulation and my period. My temper is short; I'm near tears, I am depressed. One fantastic thing – I have just discovered that I write poetry just before my period is due. I feel very creative at that time.

Best time emotionally and physically begins during menstruation. At midpoint I feel a downward shift. Most tense time is just prior to my period when physical and emotional states are at their worst. Symptoms vary from month to month.

I become a cross bitch about 4–7 days before my period, snap at my children for nothing, put down my husband, can't stand loud noise, get shaky if I have to deal with stress. My period's arrival brings me to a more optimistic frame of mind. Then, immediately after my period, it's as if I have shed something emotionally, for then I feel ready to take on some new projects, lose a couple of pounds and set new goals for myself! About midway between periods I can almost determine the moment of ovulation by a changed taste in the mouth. I now begin to crave sweet snacks until my period arrives. Naturally unusual events can obscure this pattern somewhat.

I am as witchy as hell just before the flow starts.

About a week before, my breasts seem to swell and they hurt like hell. Almost exactly seven days before I get a severe migraine which lasts a day – sometimes I throw up. . . . The symptoms haven't characterized the entire twenty-two-year span of my periods. They've occurred separately and together. The migraines were characteristic of my late teens and twenties.

A few days before my flow is to start I feel the need for extra sleep at night, and if I don't get it I become easily irritable. Also more often than not, I get a 'cleaning urge' and will clean the house, etc., with unending energy. The day I start I feel a relief and am glad the whole process is continuing okay.

What is being hypothesized about the role of men, especially husbands, in shaping, reinforcing or triggering women's perceptions and behaviour prior to menstruation? Laws (1985) has made the general case that women's perceptions and behaviour both before and during menstruation – 'menstrual etiquette' as she terms it – reflect the fact that men have long exercised power and influence to their advantage in patriarchal societies like Britain. Consider the following quotations from the studies of Lever (1980) and Shader and Ohly (1970) respectively:

As one man told me, 'I thought there was something mentally wrong with my wife. And I think she even thought she was a bit unstable. But when we realized the connection with her periods it suddenly all made sense!

Eicher makes the discerning point that the few women who do not admit to premenstrual tension are basically unaware of it, but one needs only to talk to their husbands, or co-workers, to confirm its existence.

That men frequently take the lead in defining negatively evaluated altered states or illness in women in the premenstruum is significant, in Laws's (1985b) view, because it represents a form of domination or control.

Resistance is unusual: 'Women enact their acceptance of men's definitions by complying with the etiquette' (Laws 1985a: 29). The riposte that few men either see or intend their behaviour this way is probably true, but misses the point.

Before discussing the rationale for invoking a thesis of male domination, it will be helpful briefly to address the nature of the link between the male and the medical perspective on premenstrual change. The thrust and impact of men's identification and interpretation of premenstrual change is consonant with, and legitimated by, the existence of a medical – and hence authoritative – diagnosis of premenstrual syndrome. And as was argued in chapter 2, all medical diagnoses need to be understood as social constructs, and many of them as 'man-made' social constructs. Schneider and Conrad write:

> Medical typologies are constructed primarily to redefine and solve problems presented initially in common-sense terms into medically relevant, medically manageable ones. The most significant medical typologies . . . are the diagnostic categories medical personnel use to define and structure the 'raw data' of the world as it is presented to them. They are based on the taken-for-granted meanings, assumptions, needs, and purposes dominant in contemporary medical work and their purpose is preeminently to provide a kind of order that serves subsequently as the basis for problem-solving work or 'treatment'. These medical typologies stand midway between the concrete experiences described by patients and observed clinically by physicians on the one hand, and the more abstract knowledge of medical science on the other. They are, as such, a kind of second-order typology, although importantly different from the second-order constructs the sociologist might create.
>
> (1981: 212)

One important reason why medical typologies differ from those generated by sociologists is that the latter only rarely

> enter as objects into the here-and-now experience of those studied. . . . By contrast, medical diagnoses are 'realities' with which people so designated must contend, independently of the physiological aspects of their conditions.
>
> (Schneider and Conrad 1981: 213)

Diagnoses of premenstrual syndrome constitute 'realities' which cannot be ignored and which women are predisposed through socialization – into both a negative approach to menstruation and a

Table 5.1 Symptoms associated with PMT in the medical literature

weeping	herpes	bloated feelings in
tantrums	rhinitis (runny nose)	the abdomen and
quarrels	urticaria (patches of	breasts
depression	itchy skin)	swelling in the
asthma	suicide	fingers and legs
vertigo	lethargy	increased sexual
migraine	irritability	desire
headache	dizziness	drowsiness
backache	palpitations	increased thirst or
epileptic fits	paranoid ideas	appetite
oliguria (producing	obsessive	aggression
too little urine)	compulsive	difficulty thinking in a
increase in weight	behaviour	rational way
spontaneous	impatience	forgetfulness
subcutaneous	metatarsalgia (pain in	hypersensitivity to
haemorrages	the bones of the	sounds, sight and
(bleeding under	feet)	touch
the skin)	bad breath	stimulus-overload
tightness of the	labial elephantiasis	sinusitis
clothing	(extreme	glaucoma
stiffness of the hands	enlargement of the	tension
fever	lips of the vulva)	fainting
ulcerative stomatitis	a sense of internal	exhaustion
(mouth ulcers)	shaking	upper respiratory
transient	feelings of well-being	tract infections
nymphomania	apprehension	tonsillitis
pain in the breasts	fretfulness	acne
emotional instability	sluggishness	styes
aching in the thighs	sudden outbursts of	boils
menstrual irregularity	emotion	hypoglycemia (low
nausea and vomiting	irritated eyes	blood sugar)
pruritis vulvae	reduction in hearing	hoarseness
(inflamed vulva)	or temporary	amnesia
sciatica	deafness	postural hypotension
pains in the shoulder,	bleeding from the	(low blood
knees, feet, neck	nose	pressure on
apathy	crushing chest pain	standing up
tiredness	rectal pressure	suddenly)
phobic panic attacks	feeling of pressure in	clumsiness
anger	the bladder	alcoholism
sleeplessness	hair falling out	violence
diarrhoea	muscle weakness	lack of concentration
constipation	aching and cramping	illogical reactions
feelings of intimacy	pain, swelling and	feelings of
pain	stiffness of joints	worthlessness

Source: Laws 1985b

general deference to medical expertise – to accept. And these 'realities', Laws and others would assert, are largely man-made. Table 5.1 gives a staggering list of symptoms associated with the premenstruum within the medical literature and collated by Laws (1985b: 37–8).

Laws (1985b: 35) has given clear expression to the notion of male domination or control and is worth quoting in full:

> The 'symptoms' of PMT which the doctors show most concern over – depression, anxiety and so on – are mental states which do not 'fit' with women's culturally-created notions of ourselves as nice, kind, gentle, etc. 'Mood change', as such, is often listed as a symptom – demonstrating that change *as such* is not culturally acceptable. Why *are* women's moods seen as such a problem? Men have moods too, after all. There's no evidence that women are in fact more unpredictable or inconsistent than men – it's a stereotype that men like to encourage. Couldn't it have something to do with the way that women are supposed to pander to men's moods: soothing the troubled brow, 'Did you have a good day at the office, dear?' There's just no room for women to have strong feelings of their own, disrupting this comfortable flow of emotional services.

Taylor echoes Laws:

> A double standard exists. Everyone is aware that men's moods change, but a man does not need to explain his temper tantrums and male violence is accepted as part of their nature. (The traditional wifely role was to placate men's moods.) PMS is now cited as the cause, and female frustration can continue to be ignored or invalidated; drugs are given to soothe the women and ensure they are not disruptive.
>
> (1988: 69)

Readers sceptical of such arguments should be reminded of the history of male physicians' constructions of womanhood and of 'women's disorders' sketched in chapter 2.

It is ironical that one of the most influential sponsors of the medical diagnosis of premenstrual syndrome – and of its treatment with hormone therapy – has been a female physician, Katharina Dalton (1964; 1969; 1978). A further irony is that Dalton's very approach to PMT, aimed at helping women not in a position to help themselves, affords explicit support for Laws's thesis concerning male control. She makes much of the ramifications of PMT and of hormone therapy for women's families, especially their husbands: 'many a husband has commented after the first course of injections that his wife is now more like the woman he knew at their marriage' (1969: 73). To use Shuttle and Redgrove's (1980: 51) term, Dalton emphasizes that PMT 'spreads' to others. In her controversial advocacy of the administration of progesterone for PMT, Dalton has stressed that women 'owe it to themselves and to women in general' to present for treatment; 'otherwise, they will get what they deserve from men' (quoted in Laws 1985b: 31). She instances the suffering of one husband after another as 'his darling little love bird suddenly becomes an angry, argumentative, shouting, abusive bitch' (Dalton 1978). She outlines, for example, the case of the salesman whose weekly earnings dropped by 75 per cent whenever his wife was menstruating; of the husband who asked his bank not to post the monthly statement at the usual time, which coincided with his wife's menses; and of the 40-year-old chef who was disabled with monthly attacks of bronchitis, which no treatment would alleviate until his wife's menstrual problems were addressed (quoted in Shuttle and Redgrove 1980: 51–2). As Taylor remarks, 'While Dalton is quite sincere, it is worthwhile to consider whether or not men instantly seek medical answers when they are irritable or feel violent' (1988: 62–3).

Dalton characterizes premenstrual syndrome as a temporary aberration in normally 'nice' women:

> Then suddenly her irritability ends. She is once more her usual sweet tempered and placid self, or she may be filled with guilt and remorse at the problems her actions have caused. One woman said: 'I wish others would realize that it wasn't the true me who caused all this'.
>
> (Dalton 1969: 62)

> Another pleads: 'If only you could give me something so that I'm not so spiteful against my fiancé, whom I really do love.
>
> (Dalton 1969: 111)

Several commentators have noted that women often refer to themselves as 'Jekyll and Hyde' characters, 'most of the time capable, loving and able to cope and then suddenly quite the reverse' (Lever 1980: 39). Ms N, a 39-year-old-mother participating in Scambler and Scambler's community study, saw herself in this way. She dreaded 'that week' because she knew she would be 'hateful'; and her husband, she reported, had a similar sense of foreboding: 'He doesn't like the way I feel the week beforehand because he suffers through my moods.' Her husband, 'a very good listener', had discussed her behaviour with her and had taken the initiative in suggesting she consult her general practitioner and offering to accompany her. Nobody else in the family, including Ms N's mother and her four daughters aged 18, 15, 13 and 9, was 'in the know': 'I don't feel I want to extend it to them as well: I've got to get over it!'

A summary might be helpful at this point, embracing what is *not* being argued as well as what is. It is not of course being denied here either that premenstrual change occurs or that it can be discomforting, distressing and sometimes disabling: there are occasions when premenstrual change is symptomatic of disease for which curative (or palliative) treatment may be available (see chapter 1). Nor, turning to women's husbands, is it being denied that such premenstrual change can have the effect of 'disabling the normal' (Hilbourne 1973). Finally, the claim is not being advanced that husbands and physicians are engaged in conscious conspiracies to dominate or control their wives and female patients respectively.

What, then, *is* being said? Building on themes developed in earlier chapters, it seems clear that many women are socialized into an unthinking predisposition to interpret premenstrual, and paramenstrual, change negatively. This is tapped by negatively-oriented instruments like the Moos Menstrual Distress Questionnaire, which suggest widespread symptomatology. 'Lower estimates of symptoms are obtained when data are collected prospectively and concurrently with cycle phase, and when the salience of the cycle is not apparent in the study' (Bains and Slade 1988: 469). In one recent study of nine couples who were unaware of the focus of the research, the only phase effect found was that *husbands'* 'arousal scores' increased during their wives' menses. Moreover, the day of the week was a more important factor than the menstrual cycle in determining both arousal and negative moods (Mansfield *et al.* 1989).

Historical and contemporary research on the pervasive effects of patriarchy – throughout society and within medicine – lends weight to the following wide-ranging theses:

1 Negative perceptions of menstruation in general and premenstrual syndrome or PMT in particular might plausibly be interpreted as reflecting men's domination or control over women.

2 This domination or control is most clearly articulated through the 'medicalization' of *so much* premenstrual and menstrual change, well beyond (even) medicine's own criteria of discernible pathology.

3 Both the negative evaluation and the medicalization of premenstrual and menstrual change function to preserve the asymmetrical roles of men and women in the family and in society. (No inconsistency is involved in adding that most men and most physicians would certainly take issue with this claim.)

Before elaborating on these theses through an explicit discussion of men's expressed attitudes towards menstruation, it may be instructive to close this section with a final insight from a female writer:

> might we [i.e. women] not dive deeper into menstrual pain and irritability to see what it is and use it in some positive way? In presenting this possibility, there is no intent to belittle menstrual pain or suggest it would all go away with a better attitude. Yet, some of us can benefit by looking closely at the upsets, rage, and sense of 'worthlessness' that often accompany PMS. We can ask ourselves what these worthless feelings have to say about women's position in society. If we are more sensitive and responsible in the premenstrual phase, then perhaps we realize, even unconsciously, that what bothers us is very important to us. We can't just brush it off as we usually do the rest of the month; it erupts in the classic PMS symptoms because, premenstrually, feelings we've repressed all month characteristically surface.
>
> (Taylor 1988: 70)

MENSTRUATION IN MALE CULTURE

Unfortunately, theories about men's attitudes towards menstruation are more common than empirical investigations. However, Laws (1985a) has started to make good this gap by interviewing fourteen white, well-educated men, whose ages ranged from 21 to 40, and also by recording a discussion in a 'men's group'. Much of what follows draws directly or indirectly on her pioneering work.

Laws argues that it is a mistake to put too much weight on the idea of a menstrual taboo; it is an idea which lends itself to simplistic, even misleading, analyses of cultural perspectives on menstruation. In criticism of such analyses, she writes, 'social attitudes towards menstruation are usually discussed as a set of cultural ideas, or even as an ideology, which arrives within the culture almost from outside, from above or from the past – they are disembodied "myths" ' (1985a: 13). Laws contends that it is demonstrably the case that 'male power' underpins the ubiquitous stereotypes of menstruating women apparent in patriarchal societies, but that too little attention has been paid to the construction of these stereotypes, to individual men's – frequently *ad hoc* and inconsistent – beliefs and attitudes about menstruation and how these reflect and reproduce 'male culture'. Her project is to explore what she calls an *etiquette of menstruation*, which she sees 'as part of a wider etiquette which governs the relations between women and men, marking and reinforcing each person's membership of one or other social group, and expressing their different statuses' (1985a: 13).

Laws's general argument, reminiscent of some evaluated in chapter 2, is that men maintain their power over women at least in part through 'an ideology which defines women as inferior to men, and as naturally fitting into the place men have designed for them' (1985a: 15). This dominance is expressed and reinforced by an elaborate etiquette governing relations between the sexes. Despite the fact that menstruation is not especially emphasized in western culture, male power, manifested in menstrual etiquette, inhibits women from 'generating positive self/woman-centred understandings of it for themselves' (1985a: 15).

The principal focus of her research is on 'men's talk'. Daly refers to this as 'spooking from the locker room':

> most of the time this language is used in all-male environments. Yet it is the common male view of all women and, although most women do not hear it directly, we receive it in a muted way. It is conveyed through silences, sneers, jeers, excessive politeness, paternalistic praise and disapproval, aggressive physical contact (an arm around the shoulder, a pat on the behind), invasive stares. Since women often do not *hear* the messages of obscenity directly, we are spooked. For the invasive presence and the intent are both audible and inaudible, visible and invisible.
>
> (1978: 323)

Some half of the men Laws spoke to admitted to recollections of male talk about menstruation. Boys' talk seemed most commonly to centre on jokes about sanitary towels, often resulting in the taunting of particular girls. Men's talk rarely appeared to result in taunting; rather, 'it's us and them, and they have periods, so we've got a few jokes about that sort of thing. Bit like Irish, Pakistanis . . .'.

Men's jokes characteristically focused on sexual access. One man quoted by Laws sought to distance himself from what he defined as a typical male standpoint:

> I think a lot of men will use it as a derogatory term . . . from previous experience, they'll say: 'Well she was fucking having her period, wasn't she?' Meaning they didn't have sex. 'She wasn't feeling very well', as though she did it on purpose to spite him or something. A lot of men think in those terms.

Another spoke similarly:

> When I was younger, you know, you used to say 'Oh, hard luck', kind of thing, 'picked the wrong one', that kind of thing.

As Laws (1985a: 19) remarks, this discourse defines women both as existing solely for men's sexual use, and as essentially interchangeable in their sexual relation to men; a man may 'pick the wrong one'.

Laws asked why menstruation never featured in the pornography that one man explained was regularly exchanged in his work place. She was told that men did not find it erotic, and also that one simply did not have sex during menstruation. The same man told the following story about his boss at work:

> there was a female toilet just outside the lab so we could always see the women going to the toilet, and he actually used to time them, and if they were taking a long time he used to say, 'Oh well, they've got the rags up, there's no point in chatting her up.'

Weideger suggests that norms forbidding sexual intercourse during menstruation have been common throughout history and across cultures. She goes on to describe a study utilizing menstrual questionnaires with 960 families in California. It was found that half the men and women abstained from intercourse during menstruation. Twenty-five per cent of the women said that they objected to intercourse during menses, while 41 per cent said that male partners occasionally or frequently objected to sex at 'that time of the month' (Weideger 1975: 126).

Paige (1973) hypothesized that women who had a lighter flow while using contraceptive pills would be less likely to object to sexual intercourse than women whose flow had remained unchanged and was relatively heavy. To put this hypothesis to the test, she studied 52 women, all married and all on the contraceptive pill. Fifty-five per cent of the women in the study did not have sex during menstruation. When abstinence was correlated with amount of flow, however, Paige found that 62 per cent of those with normal flow did not engage in sex during menstruation, while only 35 per cent of those with light flow abstained. She concluded that women who have less menstrual 'mess' have less allegiance to the putative taboo against menstrual sex.

But Weideger suggests a rival thesis: 'Might the women in Paige's study who had less of the "mess" of menstruation appear to be relatively free from the taboo because their *partners*, and not the *women*, were less frequently repulsed by menstruation?' (1975: 127). Elaborating on this thesis, she argues that to the extent that women are swayed by men's opinions, the male response to menstruation will affect the way women feel about sexual activity. She continues,

Abstinence from sex during menstruation, whatever its component motives, supports and reinforces the menstrual taboo and confirms the belief that there is something wrong with menstruating women – something that makes sexual activity unappealing. . . . The presence of menstrual shame combined with sexual hibernation during flow corroborates the view that women are in fact less sexual than men. After all, if she cannot, or will not, have sex for a quarter of her life during the fertile years, she is 'clearly' less sexual.

(1975: 128)

It is a complex, even tortuous, argument, resting on the premiss that while it is men rather than women who find sex during menstruation unappealing, men typically hold women culpable for denying them sexual access (see also Laws (1985a) below).

In the previous chapter it was noted that Scambler and Scambler found that 16 per cent of the women who reported periods diminishing the quality of their lives specified an adverse effect on their sex lives. In the same study the total sample of 79 women were asked if they ever had sexual intercourse during their menses. Eighteen per cent replied that they did on occasion; 1 per cent, one woman, said that she had done so, but only when her flow was particularly light; and the remaining 81 per cent answered that they had never had intercourse during menstruation. The high proportion – relative to those in the American studies – denying ever having had sex during menses may possibly be explicable in terms of the social composition of the sample, four out of every five coming from working-class households (Scambler and Scambler 1986).

Sexuality apart, Laws draws attention to two other themes of men's talk about menstruation. The first is that women 'use' it to get out of things. Laws quotes a man making this point in relation to menstrual pain:

I can remember that that was often a male reaction to period pains, that it was something that was completely not understandable, that it was something that was, that shouldn't happen, so therefore, men tended to think that it didn't happen, that it was something that women made up, to get out of things. I can remember feeling irritated, feeling annoyed, feeling that there was nothing . . . that I didn't have any control over the situation, and that it was something that women used to exert control.

(1985a: 20–1)

And second, the men who spoke to Laws communicated the idea that the menstrual cycle somehow makes women moody, bad-tempered and unreliable. 'Often this was referred to as "the time of the month", which makes it unnecessary to be exact about *which* time of the month is meant' (1985a: 20). Laws asked one man if the women he worked with ever mentioned their periods.

> No, but it usually became evident. . . . Because of, er well, whether it was actually evident or whether it was an imagined, imagined that it was, like they were in a bad mood and I think you imagined it because it was their period. . . . Because mainly in my job, it tended to be the women that did it, I was always in a minority, either on my own or with one or two others. And so if there were a lot of women there'd obviously be someone who was in a bad mood because they were menstruating, at least that's what we put it down to.

> It was not discussed with the women. Um, maybe sometimes we'd overhear women saying, 'Oh, she's in a bad mood, but it's that time of the month', so they'd sort of forgive her. . . . But I think it was mainly to do with the men. And even, maybe because I'd worked with other men and we'd talk around that, that you know: 'Oh, she's in a bad mood, she's bloody menstruating again' . . . when I worked on my own with women I still had that mentality, that you know: 'Jesus Christ, who's menstruating again?'

> (1985a: 21)

Laws refers to this kind of joking within men's talk as 'policing the periphery'.

ASPECTS OF MENSTRUAL ETIQUETTE

Using the insights gleaned from often uneasy and awkward discussions with men about 'men's talk' and menstruation, Laws returns to the issue of menstrual etiquette. Several aspects of her discussion are worth highlighting here. First, the 'rule behind all the others' seems to be that women are not permitted to draw men's attention to menstruation. This is especially true in the public domain; in private, men – husbands in particular – may of course agree to waive the rules. Laws was struck, however, by how few men had ever heard their mothers or sisters discuss menstruation. As adults many remained deeply uncomfortable if, for example, they saw packets of sanitary towels or Tampax lying around.

> One of the big surprises of adult life was going into people's houses and finding things openly displayed in places. I couldn't believe it, because at home these things had always been hidden away, and it was

a real shock to me, because it was like something that was not mentioned, never spoken about.

(Laws 1985a: 24)

Laws points out that men's sense of 'what is due to them as men' is offended by women not properly observing the etiquette of concealment.

Second, Laws argues that women must assume that menstruation is actually offensive to men, and behave accordingly, unless given explicit permission to assume otherwise. As discussed in the last section, men often seem to define sex during menstruation as undesirable or forbidden. It was apparently acceptable, however, for men, if not for women, to initiate sexual activity during periods. Laws writes, 'When they talked about sex during periods, what seemed to interest them was breaking rules, not ignoring them or doing away with them.' Thus:

> I think I thought it was . . . no, not dirty . . . I think I thought that it was exciting, you know, that we were sort of breaking some rule . . . that particular rule was broken along with a whole lot of other rules at the same time . . . it developed in terms of what I was thinking about things in general.

And another:

> Yes it rings bells,yes. . . . It does for me . . . but like we talked about it before, for me at least part of it is to do with the unacceptability of periods, right from being little . . . I mean that was all sorts of things. Like touching or looking at, well anybody's genitals, it wasn't on . . . and that makes the idea of doing so quite interesting. And periods were really sort of beyond the pale, you know, that's almost a last barrier in not-allowed behaviour, which is now OK, and I think that adds an extra . . . it's forbidden fruit, I think.

(1985a: 26)

A third, related, point is that this issue of sex during menstruation was *the* issue about menstruation for many men, which, as Laws notes, puts 'the whole experience into a sexual context which is not the context women tend to see it in' (1985a: 27). Indeed, 'the sexualization of menstruation becomes a problem in itself'.

To summarize Laws's account: she sees current cultural attitudes towards menstruation as 'part of the process by which men maintain their social power over women'. For her, male culture generates and enforces 'male-supremacist definitions of menstruation'. In her own words,

Etiquette is one procedure by which women's compliance with these definitions is policed. Hiding the existence of periods forces women to be endlessly aware of men's potential presence, their gaze entering even the most private and mundane parts of a woman's life. And, if women may not speak in public about periods, they are blocked from generating new understandings of their bodies which could challenge men's.

(1985a: 29)

We return to the thesis of men's domination or control over women in the final chapter. It seems appropriate to end this one with a brief reference to a calculatingly polemical piece by Gloria Steinem (1984) called 'If men could menstruate'. Steinem gives a long, amusing and potent list of consequences 'if suddenly, magically, men could menstruate and women could not'. The list begins:

Clearly, menstruation would become an enviable, boast-worthy, masculine event:

Men would brag about how long and how much.

Young boys would talk about it as the envied beginning of manhood. Gifts, religious ceremonies, family dinners, and stag parties would mark the day.

To prevent monthly work loss among the powerful, Congress would fund a National Institute of Dysmenorrhoea. Doctors would research little about heart attacks, from which men were hormonally protected, but everything about cramps.

Sanitary supplies would be federally funded and free.

(1984: 338)

And so on. Steinem's contention is that 'logic is in the eye of the logician'. If, she posits in her concluding paragraph, women are supposed to be less rational and more emotional at the commencement of their menstrual cycle, then why is it not logical to say that, in those few days, 'women behave the most like the way men behave all month long'? 'The truth is', she adds, 'that if men could menstruate, the power justifications would go on and on' (1984: 340).

Chapter 6

Menstrual change and social and work activity

Menstrual change can impinge upon and occasionally disrupt women's lives outside as well as inside the home. In the first part of this chapter the focus is on menstrual change in relation to school and work. There is a discussion of how to interpret the links frequently postulated in the medical and academic literature between periods, period problems, absenteeism and diminished work performance. Attention is paid also to the coping strategies adopted by girls and women in the face of self- or other-defined obstacles to working through menstrual change. This is followed by a brief review of analyses of menses and sporting activity.

The second part of the chapter is a consideration of the advantages and disadvantages of the use of premenstrual or menstrual change to absolve women from responsibility for their actions. This features a discussion of recent legal cases involving premenstrual syndrome.

Finally, there is an examination of the complex interrelationships between biographical disruption, life events, distress and disorder directly associated with the menstruum. This incorporates a review and analysis of the nature of the alleged link between minor psychiatric disorder and menstrual phenomena. Emphasis is given, as elsewhere, to the pitfalls and problems of interpreting available data that bear on these issues.

MENSTRUAL CHANGE AND WORK ACTIVITY

Studies on menstrual pain in adolescent girls have shown prevalences ranging from 13 per cent to 80 per cent or more (Teperi and Rimpela 1989). Much of this variation is explicable in terms of methodological factors, like sampling strategies, and the differing criteria of pain used. According to Teperi and Rimpela's review of the literature, a substantial proportion of girls have menstrual pain during the first year after

Table 6.1 Socio-epidemiological studies on menstrual pain among adolescent girls

Study	Sample (Number)	Main findings
Miller	Young college women and nurses, USA (785)	47% have dysmenorrhoea; 17% need bed rest
Heald *et al.*	High school girls, mostly aged 16–17.5, USA (392)	21% absent from school at least once a year; 19% have asked a physician for help
Golub *et al.*	Philadelphia high school girls (16,183)	33% frequent dysmenorrhoea; 33% occasional dysmenorrhoea
Widholm and Kantero	Finnish school girls aged 10–20 (8,111)	Prevalence grows in the years after menarche: 36% (1st year) to 72% (5–9 yr)
Timonen and Procope	Finnish university students (748)	Physical activity in negative correlation to menstrual pain
Widholm	Finnish school girls aged 13–20 (331)	23% miss school
Klein and Litt	US probability sample girls aged 12–17 (2,699)	25% of excessive school absences due to menstrual pain; increasing prevalence by increasing gynaecological age/Tanner stage; SES positively correlated to menstrual pain
Svanberg and Ulmsten	Swedish school girls aged 10–19 (502)	9% stay in bed; 23% use drugs; 25% limit normal activities
Andersch and Milsom	Random sample, women aged 19 of Gothenburg (656)	8% stay at home during every menstruation; use of tobacco negatively correlated to menstrual pain

Source: Teperi and Rimpela 1989

menarche, prevalence then increases with age, and 'the majority of girls experience at least some pain a few years after menarche' (1989: 163). In one Swedish sample of 19-year-old girls, approximately 40 per cent regularly took medication for menstrual pain (Andersch and Milsom 1982). Menstrual pain, Teperi and Rimpela add, whether or not formally diagnosed as dysmenorrhea, frequently disrupts activity and is often cited as one of the major causes of school absenteeism among adolescent girls. Studies bearing this out are summarized in Table 6.1.

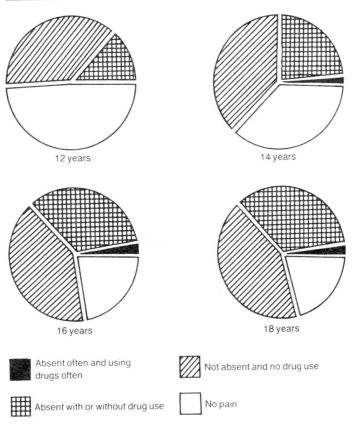

Figure 6.1 Menstrual pain, use of medication and absenteeism, in post-menarcheal girls aged 12, 14, 16 and 18

Source: Teperi and Rimpela 1989

Teperi and Rimpela conducted their own study, using postal questionnaires with a sample consisting of all girls born on consecutive days in July 1964, 1966, 1968 and 1970, in Finland. The post-menarcheal girls were asked whether they had experienced severe, mild or no menstrual pain, whether they had taken medication to relieve menstrual pain, and whether they had stayed at home because of pain during the previous six months. All indicators of menstrual pain showed an increase with age. Approximately half the 12-year-old post-menarcheal girls reported at least mild menstrual pain, compared with 80 per cent of the 18-year-olds. The prevalence of severe pain quadrupled over the same period of time.

Use of medication and absenteeism owing to menstrual pain was found to correlate with the severity of pain. For example, among the 16-year-old girls reporting severe pain, 69 per cent had resorted to medication and 54 per cent had remained at home during the previous six months, while 24 per cent had used medication and 15 per cent had stayed at home among those reporting mild pain. The authors point out that some commentators, for example Ylikorkala and Dawood (1978), have proposed that 'the term dysmenorrhoea would be justified if a woman seeks relief for her pain from a physician or by self-medication' (1989: 166). Figure 6.1 presents the data on menstrual pain, use of medication and absenteeism in post-menarcheal girls aged 12, 14, 16 and 18 in Finland.

In all age groups the majority of girls disclosed at least mild menstrual pain during the previous six months. Approximately 10 per cent in the youngest age group, and nearly 40 per cent in the two oldest ones, had experienced pain sufficiently severe to compel them to stay at home or use drugs, or both, at least once during the same period. In Finland, Teperi and Rimpela conclude, 'thousands of young girls are markedly incapacitated by menstrual pain'. They add, however, that menstrual pain is not the most significant cause of school absenteeism: 'respiratory tract diseases were 2-3 times more prevalent causes of absenteeism when compared with menstrual pain in various age groups of girls' (1989: 167).

Consistent with these results are the various claims that pain or other forms of menstrual change frequently reduce the efficiency of children and adults at school and work respectively, either through absenteeism or diminished performance. Dalton (1960) claimed to have found that among girls in an English boarding school infractions such as unpunctuality, forgetfulness and the avoidance of games were about twice as common during menstruation as would be expected had they been evenly distributed throughout the cycle. She has additionally claimed empirical support for the proposition that girls' performance in school examinations is affected detrimentally by menstruation (1968).

Dalton is also the key exponent of the view that amongst adult women the cost to industry of menstrual problems is high. She continues,

> It has been estimated to cost British industry 3 per cent of its total wage bill, which may be compared with 3 per cent in Italy, 5 per cent in Sweden and 8 per cent in America. The load is not spread evenly, for the industries which suffer most are those employing large numbers of women, especially the clothing industry, light engineering, transistor and assembly factories and laundries.

Absenteeism due to problems associated with the menstruum she attributes mainly to spasmodic dysmenorrhoea, premenstrual migraine and asthma. Predictably, she sees premenstrual syndrome as the principal cause of work disruption, if not of absenteeism. As one library assistant told her, 'You don't stay away from work merely because of your bad temper, instead you soldier on and cause chaos by misfiling, and you get yourself a bad name' (1978: 114).

The following lengthy quotation reveals the extent of Dalton's commitment to the thesis that menstrual change has a pernicious effect on work:

> The lowering of mental ability during the paramenstruum accounts for unnecessary typing errors and more than one secretary has been referred for treatment when her boss could no longer put up with those few days in each month when letters had to be returned for retyping. Journalists, artists and authors find this a problem too, lacking inspiration and waiting hopefully for a brainwave, which is more likely to come during the postmenstruum. Errors of billing, accounts, stock-taking and filing take longer to correct than to perform, and again the incidence of mistakes is highest during the paramenstruum. Premenstrual irritability may show itself in bad-tempered service by shopworkers, receptionists and waitresses, who are in the public eye. Lowered judgement during the premenstruum must also be considered by teachers, magistrates and examiners. Hasty and wrong decisions are the problems of executives. One teacher wrote with honesty, 'Every month there are one or two days when I am simply not worth the salary my employers pay me.'
>
> (Dalton 1978: 115–16)

Premenstrual syndrome, according to Dalton, can affect women's chances of getting a job, holding it down, receiving promotion and losing it unnecessarily.

Lever's (1980) popular text on premenstrual syndrome includes several quotations from women struggling to find work or cope when there:

> I have to find a job and I'm extremely worried about the timing of the hoped-for interviews, because in the week before my period my ability to present myself diminishes sharply. Apart from a general appearance of unassertiveness, I can go totally blank or burst into tears. I know I always manage one way or another, but it is dreadful feeling so impotent.

Often it was all I could do not to scream 'leave me alone' and throw all my papers in the air as I ran crying from the room. But somehow, I'd manage to hang on. I'd try to avoid meetings and postpone important decision making during my premenstrual week, but of course that was not always possible.

I get very irritable before my periods, but obviously I can't afford to let this show too much at work, particularly when interviewing someone on the air. So I bite back my irritation as much as I can during the day and shamelessly take it out on my long-suffering partner when I get home. I hate myself for being like this but each month, no matter how hard I try, the same thing happens. Sometimes it makes my work a tremendous strain and I have to admit that it does suffer then. But I think I make up for that by the extra energy I put into it during the rest of the month.

(Lever 1980: 85–8)

This association between premenstrual and menstrual change and lowered productivity or job disruption has been questioned by a number of authors. Some have aptly queried the methodology and manner of interpretation of data in the investigations of Dalton and others (Parlee 1973); and some have failed to find the association (e.g. Golub 1976). But some critics have gone further. Martin suggests that it is highly significant that when Frank (1931) identified premenstrual syndrome immediately after the Depression he discussed it in relation to women's capacity to work. It was a time when women were coming under increasing pressure to give up waged work in favour of men. Can it be accidental, Martin asks, that numerous studies were published in the interwar years that showed the debilitating effects of menstruation on work? Predictably, she continues, when women were required for the labour force during the Second World War, 'a rash of studies found that menstruation was not a liability after all' (Martin 1989: 120). And when, after the Second World War, women were again displaced from many of the paid jobs they had taken on, there was once more 'a spate of menstrual research' showing that 'women were indeed disabled by their hormones'. She notes that research conducted by Dalton in the 1940s was published in the *British Medical Journal* in 1953; and Dalton, as we have seen, was, and is, at pains to emphasize the economic and social costs of premenstrual syndrome.

Martin's hypothesis, then, is that it is when women's participation in the labour force is seen as a threat that data and theories addressing the negative effects of menstrual change, particularly on 'activities involving mental or physical discipline', feature in the public domain. She argues that this perception of threat has never been more apparent than since the mid-1970s. (Laws (1985), in similar vein, has suggested that the recent burgeoning of emphasis on premenstrual syndrome might also be interpreted as a response to 'the second wave of feminism'.) Martin goes on to argue that, with respect to the increasingly routine and de-skilled employment available in late industrial societies like the USA and Britain, the bulk of the population, including all but a very few women, are now subject to strict mental and physical work discipline; this is one manifestation of what Foucault calls a 'micro-physics of power', 'small acts of cunning' in the total enterprise of producing 'docile bodies' (1979). What many women seem to report is that they are, during premenstrual days, less willing or able to tolerate such discipline' (Martin 1989: 122).

Indeed, many premenstrual symptoms seem to focus on intolerance of the kind of discipline required for 'the increasingly routine and de-skilled' work inside as well as outside the home. Consider the following statement by Dalton:

> Then quite suddenly you feel as if you can't cope any more – everything seems too much trouble, the endless household chores, the everlasting planning of meals. For no apparent reason you rebel: 'Why should I do everything?' you ask defiantly. 'I didn't have to do this before I was married. Why should I do it now?' . . . As on other mornings you get up and cook breakfast while your husband is in the bathroom. You climb wearily out of bed and trudge down the stairs, a vague feeling of resentment growing within you. The sound of cheerful whistling from upstairs only makes you feel a little more cross. Without any warning the toast starts to scorch and the sausages instead of happily sizzling in the pan start spitting and spluttering furiously. Aghast you rescue the toast which by this time is beyond resurrection and fit only for the trash. The sausages are charred relics of their former selves and you throw those out too. Your unsuspecting husband opens the kitchen door expecting to find his breakfast ready and waiting, only to see a smoky atmosphere and a thoroughly overwrought wife. You are so dismayed at him finding you in such chaos that you just burst helplessly into tears.

Needless to say, Dalton's solution is the seeking of professional medical help, usually treatment with progesterone (see chapter 5). As Martin comments, 'the content of the women's remarks, the substance of what she objects to, escape notice' (1989: 125).

A number of the women interviewed by Martin and her colleagues gave expression to the double message that women workers receive in relation to premenstrual syndrome. One is worth quoting at length:

> Something I hear a lot that really amazes me is that women are discriminated against because they get their period. It makes them less capable to do certain kinds of work. It makes me angry. I never faced it in terms of my own personal experience, but it's something I've heard. I grew up thinking you shouldn't draw attention to your period, it makes you seem less capable than a man. I always tried to be a kind of a martyr, and then all of a sudden recently I started hearing all this scientific information that shows that women really do have a cycle that affects their mood, and they really do get into bad moods when they have their periods. I don't know whether all of a sudden it gives legitimacy to start complaining that it's okay. I think I have a hard time figuring out what that's supposed to do. Then again you can look at that as being a really negative thing, medical proof that women are less reliable. It's proven now that they're going to have bad moods once a month and not be as productive.
>
> (Martin 1989: 127)

Martin suggests that the way out of this 'bind' may be to focus on 'women's experiential statements', and what many women say is that they function differently during certain days, in ways that render them intolerant of the discipline required of them by work. 'We could then perhaps hear these statements not as warnings of the flaws inside women that need to be fixed but as insights into flaws in society that need to be addressed' (1989: 127).

COPING AT WORK

Because women are typically socialized into thinking of menstruation negatively, as a phenomenon to be hidden, it becomes a 'hassle' in public places: nobody must witness the mechanics of coping with 'mess'. School and work environments may present special problems. 'The "hassle" refers to the host of practical difficulties involved in getting through the day of menstruating, given the way our time and space are organized in schools and places of work' (Martin 1989: 93). How, for example, does the girl at school find time and private space to change pads or tampons?

> In school it's hard; teachers don't want to let you out of the classroom, they're upset if you're late and give you a hard time.

In the seventh grade I didn't even carry a pocketbook or anything – wow! – how do you stash a maxi-pad in your notebook and try to get to the bathroom between classes to change? It was like a whole procedure, to make sure nobody saw, that none of the guys saw. From your notebook and into your pocket or take your whole notebook to the ladies' room which looks absolutely ridiculous.

Few work environments are any more conducive to women with periods: 'I have to go to the bathroom more often, and because I work with two men I can't just say "oops" and go.'

One woman told of an 'excruciating incident' on her first day delivering goods to several small stores, accompanied by her boss. As well as needing frequent visits to the toilet she had severe cramps: 'I couldn't even tell him, because that stuff isn't spoken of, what the matter was with me' (1989: 93–4). These recollections from Martin's study in the USA nicely complement Laws's explication of male culture and menstrual etiquette discussed in chapter 5.

Martin stresses that the girl pondering how to sneak a tampon from the classroom to the bathroom, and the woman who feels she cannot tell her boss what is wrong, are being invited to do the impossible: 'conceal and control their bodily functions in institutions whose organization of time and space take little cognizance of them'. This invitation to 'do the impossible' may still be routinely extended, but Martin insists that women should not merely be characterized as passive victims of an ideology that demeans them. She suggests, for example, that the toilet or bathroom – the place that women use to take care of their bodily functions, including menstruation – constitutes a

complex backstage area in contrast to the school, factory, or firm's public front stage area. Contemporary women students or workers can use bathrooms not only as places to keep their menstrual blood from showing but as places to preserve a bit of autonomy and room for themselves in a context where their physical movements are often rigidly controlled.

(Martin 1989: 94)

Moreover, useable backstage areas, more or less taken for granted nowadays although rare a century ago, also afford women opportunities in management's time to debate and conspire against aspects of management policy (Shapiro-Peel 1984).

Brief opportunities to be subversive may seem poor compensation for a multiplicity of obstacles to coping with menstrual change in public places like schools, factories and offices. Dalton has made a point of stressing that convenient facilities need to be made available for women in public places. She also commends the extension of flexitime. More controversially, she adds,

> perhaps industry should tackle the problem more seriously by educating its staff, especially personnel managers and forewomen, to recognize and fully understand the problems so that women can be assigned to less skilled jobs, such as packing and stacking, during their vulnerable days rather than remaining on tasks which are harder to remedy later, such as soldering or filing.
>
> (1978: 119–20)

Any qualms about this unthinking sexism aside, there remain difficulties about the institutionalization of 'excusing conditions' for menstrual change. These difficulties are addressed below, with particular reference to the law.

MENSES AND SPORTING ACTIVITY

Dalton's (1960) claim that girls in a boarding school tended to avoid games during menstruation probably reflects an understandable psychological inhibition on their part rather than any anticipated effect on performance. In fact, after a comprehensive review of the published literature on menstruation and sporting activity, Wells states,

> there is no conclusive evidence to suggest that menstrual function affects physical performance. With a few exceptions (for example, in women with serious dysmenorrhoea), physical performance is *not* altered by menstrual phase. Possibly there is a phase of the cycle in which a particular athlete may be more or less efficient, but the differences are so small that in daily performance they are not noticeable.
>
> (1985: 77)

For elite women athletes, however, these slight variations in efficiency may be of more significance; and some may be more keenly 'tuned' to such variations than others. Wells opposes the use of oral contraceptives to alter the menstrual cycle to fit an athlete's performance schedule, suggesting that the well-documented side-effects of the pill may more seriously threaten athletic performance than would the normal menstrual cycle (1985: 105). She also notes that, while 'for some women (and maybe all), juxtaposing the menstrual cycle and training schedule to plan when workouts are to be most strenuous, when "peaking" is to be achieved, and when rest is needed may be extremely important in maximizing performance' (1985: 77), it remains the case that women have become Olympic champions and set world records during all phases, including menstruation.

PREMENSTRUAL SYNDROME OR PMT AND THE LAW

The question as to whether change associated with the menstruum might relieve a woman of full responsibility for those of her actions committed in the course of that change has been hotly debated, perhaps most dramatically in relation to two recent legal cases. Early in 1980 a woman called Sandie Smith, who had a protracted history of recurrent violent behaviour, stabbed and killed a colleague after an argument at work. She was tried and eventually found guilty, not of murder, but of manslaughter due to diminished responsibility, her sentence being a period of probation under medical supervision. The following day a second woman, Christine English, who had killed her lover by running him down with a car, was similarly found not guilty of murder but guilty of manslaughter due to diminished responsibility: she was conditionally discharged without punishment. The link in these two cases was that in each a decisive factor in determining lenient sentencing was the acceptance of medical testimony, involving Dalton, that the crimes had been perpetrated while the women were suffering from severe symptoms of premenstrual syndrome (Allen 1990: 200).

On the face of it these judgements represented a positive move towards women's equality. After all, and some would protest not before time, they seemed to embody an acknowledgement of the medical reality of premenstrual syndrome and of its capacity to temporarily induce 'diminished responsibility'. As Allen recounts, however, these legal judgements provoked considerable unease. The unease concerned the possible implications of the judgements. Squire wrote:

> The medical evidence on which both cases relied made these two women particular examples of a condition from which, it claimed, all women suffer to some extent. Implicitly, all women who menstruate are at times not responsible for their actions, are close to madness and prone to crime.
>
> (1981: 16)

It is not necessary, however, to believe that premenstrual syndrome is a universal female problem in order to see that the special treatment given to Sandie Smith and Christine English has major implications for women, both within the system of criminal justice and elsewhere. Allen takes one of the lower estimated rates for premenstrual syndrome amongst women – 25 per cent – and offers the following calculations:

> a straightforward calculation will reveal that at any one time about one in every sixteen women of menstrual age will be both a sufferer of the condition and currently in the relevant phase of her cycle. On this basis, even if there were no statistical correlation between menstrual phase and crime, one in sixteen female offenders in this age group could legitimately claim, by reference to these precedents, that she had grounds for special treatment because of the psychological disruptions caused by her condition.
>
> (1990: 210)

She adds that if these figures are compared to their equivalents for the most common psychological disorders routinely taken into account as possible grounds for such special treatment – for example, depression (one in 30), or schizophrenia (one in 100) – 'it should be clear that the acceptance of premenstrual tension as a legally relevant disorder affecting 25% of women 25% of the time would be likely to have major legal consequences' (1990: 210). First, it would presumably herald a major increase in the number of cases in which mental abnormality would be judged relevant to legal decision-making, and therefore in the number of instances in which physicians became involved in the criminal process. Second, since this increase would pertain entirely to women, it would result in a highly significant increase in the '(already existing) sexual *disparity* in the deployment of medical and psychiatric evidence in legal actions'. And third, as a corollary, it would lead to an overall change in the sentencing of women offenders, with a marked reduction in severe and custodial sentences and an increase in women receiving compulsory medical treatment.

Allen notes that these implications of the Smith and English judgements were quickly criticized, but from two very different perspectives. Some were afraid that premenstrual syndrome would become a woman's 'all-purpose excuse', which, as Laws stresses, echoes an important theme in 'male culture's version of menstruation' (1990: 205) (see chapter 5). Christine English's lawyer fuelled such fears when he admitted after the trial that he had hit upon this possible line of defence 'very much by serendipity and pursued it merely on the strength of the coincidence of Ms English's crime with her premenstruum (rather than any clear medical history of premenstrual disorder)' (Allen 1990: 211).

The second critical response to the implication of the two cases arose from a concern that the acceptance of premenstrual syndrome as a natural weakness of the female constitution might undermine women's claims for sexual equality. Some feminists felt, consistently with arguments by Laws and others reported in the last chapter, that acceptance of these legal decisions could reinforce an ideological conception of women as inherently irresponsible or unstable. More directly,

> it was felt that through their acceptance of what might be seen as an inherent female tendency toward cyclical instability and incapacity, these cases might provide a specific legal precedent by which to justify discriminatory treatment of women in employment, education, political life, and so on.
>
> (Allen 1990: 211)

A number of employers in the USA have argued against the employment of women for certain posts using precisely these grounds. To make the point in the most general way, the more common and acceptable it becomes to explicate premenstrual and menstrual change in terms of medically defined 'disease', the more common and acceptable it may be to confine women to the private domain by discriminating against them in significant sectors of the public domain. For example, to legitimate absence from school or work too readily in accordance with often irrational diagnoses of menorrhagia, dysmenorrhoea or premenstrual syndrome by physicians (who are usually male) would in effect be to confirm women as inferior to, and uncompetitive with, men in the public domain. The issue of generating consensus on an 'appropriate balance' here is taken up in chapter 7.

Another related argument advanced by feminists concerns the 'medicalization' of female deviance. Squire (1981) has claimed that accounting for women's crimes or deviant behaviour in terms of medical conditions 'puts women down'; it deprives them of responsibility for their actions and leaves them under the essentially patriarchal control of the medical profession. Allen writes, 'the medical approach aligns conformity with health and deviance with disease, and there is no reason to suppose that in relation to premenstrual "deviance" it would restrict itself to criminal matters' (1990: 211). She quotes Dalton's 'heavily normative remarks' in support of this view:

> Amongst PMS women increased libido is occasionally noticed in the premenstruum. . . . All too often it is this nymphomanic urge in adolescents which is responsible for young girls running away from

home, or custody, only to be found wandering in the park or following the boys. These girls can be helped, and their criminal career abruptly ended with hormone therapy.

(Dalton 1982: 94)

There is certainly an irony in focusing on the *problem* of girls 'following the boys'. To hark back to Steinem's 'If men could menstruate' (1984), what of boys who spend many of their conscious hours, all month long, following the girls? Do they similarly require biomedical therapy? We return to the complex of issues about menstrual change and gender relations discussed in this and the preceding chapter in the final chapter of this text.

BIOGRAPHICAL DISRUPTION AND MENSTRUAL CHANGE

If menstrual change can lead to biographical disruption, so can biographical disruption lead to premenstrual and menstrual change. Passing references were made to this possibility in the brief review of the medical literature in chapter 1. In this section we focus on the possible aetiological role of both significant life events and psychiatric symptomatology in premenstrual and menstrual change.

There has long been evidence that life events marking sharp and threatening disruptions or transitions in women's lives can lead to menstrual irregularity (Harris 1989). During the Second World War, for example, Sydenham (1946) reported that only 35 per cent of women held in Stanley Camp, Honk Kong, retained regular menstruation. Fifty-four per cent experienced amenorrhoea for longer than three months. Bass (1947) reported an incidence of secondary amenorrhoea among 800 women in a concentration camp at Theresienstadt, ranging from 25 per cent among those aware that they were to stay for a protracted period to 54 per cent among those aware that they were passing through *en route* for an unknown destination (i.e., who were in a situation even more fraught with uncertainty and threat). Secondary amenorrhoea generally appeared within two months of incarceration, when anxiety was probably at its peak. This promptness of onset led to the differentiation of such 'psychogenic amenorrhoea' from that due to malnutrition, which eventually caused amenorrhoea in nine out of ten detained women.

Since these pioneering studies, far less threatening life events than wartime incarceration have been implicated in menstrual change. One of the most systematic of recent studies is Harris's (1989) investigation of 65 women with secondary amenorrhoea, 98 with menorrhagia and 224 in a comparison group. The possible causal role of a number of factors, including life events and psychiatric symptomatology, was examined. According to Harris, the two conditions under investigation showed contrasting patterns, in relation to both the type of life stress preceding them, and the intervening psychiatric symptoms. She summarizes as follows:

> It appeared that provoking agents (especially those involving loss) and depression were involved over quite some months in many onsets of menorrhagia; by contrast, secondary amenorrhoea appeared to be preceded by challenge experiences within a very recent period, and there also seemed to be some role for intervening tension or fatigue.
>
> (Harris 1989: 284)

On the basis of these findings Harris proffers some speculations. One of these is that there may be a so far unmeasured predisposition to react to challenges in a way that contributes to secondary amenorrhoea; and she goes on to cite Shanan and colleagues' (1965) reference to someone with a 'strong striving to demonstrate independence by active involvement' as a candidate for such a predisposition. She recalls one of her own interviewees' accounts of reaction to threat:

> One girl, for example, threw herself into nursing her mentally deranged mother, while gritting her teeth with determination not to be hurt. And certainly the low rate of onset of psychiatric disorder among the secondary amenorrhoea women would be consistent with the notion of their protecting themselves against such anxieties, with the tension and fatigue states perhaps forming part of such an effort at suppression.
>
> (1989: 285)

Harris also hypothesizes that the high rate of secondary amenorrhoea found among elite athletes may not be wholly explicable in terms of the somatic effects of prolonged exercise, as generally assumed, but may additionally involve attributes of challenge and dedication.

Turning to menorrhagia, Harris notes that reports of menstrual blood loss are notoriously unreliable (see chapter 1). She wonders, in fact, if 'the role of provoking agents and depression may be to increase psychic reactivity to menstrual blood loss rather than to increase blood loss itself' (1989: 289). Sensibly and understandably she emphasizes just how tentatively her hypotheses are framed and the continuing need for further empirical work.

A number of other more general studies have examined possible relationships between minor psychiatric symptomatology and self-reported symptoms associated with the menstruum. One such study was carried out by Scambler and Scambler (1986) with a community sample of 79 women. The women were visited twice in their homes. On the first occasion they were briefly interviewed, filled in the 30-item General Health Questionnaire (GHQ) (Goldberg 1972), and were given and advised about completion of six-week health diaries. The second visit occurred at the end of the health diary period. The women were then interviewed in detail about their diary entries, their perceptions and past and present experiences of menstrual disorders and any medical treatment received for them. And finally, they completed a shortened version of the Moos Menstrual Distress Questionnaire (MMDQ) (see chapter 4).

The mean item score on the 30-item GHQ was 3.9, with a range of 0–19. Seventy per cent of the women had a score of four or less and were classified as GHQ negative (GHQ–). The remaining 30 per cent had a score of five or more and were classified as GHQ positive (GHQ+). The GHQ+ figure of 30 per cent is higher than that reported in some other community-based studies. Goldberg and his colleagues (1976), for example, found that only 16 per cent of a random sample of women were GHQ+. The high rate in Scambler and Scambler's study is almost certainly a function of the socio-demographic characteristics of the sample (Goldberg and Huxley 1980; Scambler and Scambler 1986).

The symptoms most frequently reported as distressing during the premenstruum and during flow, and the manner of their calculation on the basis of completion of the shortened version of the MMDQ, have been described in some detail in chapter 4. As far as the premenstruum is concerned, 72 per cent of women registered at least one distressing symptom. Eighty-seven per cent of those with GHQ+ status registered distressing symptoms, compared with 65 per cent of those with GHQ– status (p<0.05). The former recorded a mean of 4.7 distressing symptoms, the latter a mean of 2.4. Table 6.2 gives the rank order of the 12 symptoms most frequently defined as distressing during the premenstruum. It can be seen that four of these were significantly associated with GHQ+ status: depression, irritability, headaches and anxiety. Six of the remaining eight items also showed a positive, if not statistically significant, association with GHQ+ status.

Sixty-seven per cent reported one or more distressing symptoms during menstrual flow. Once again, there was a significant positive association with GHQ+ status: 83 per cent of those with GHQ+ status reported distressing symptoms, compared with 60 per cent of those with GHQ– status (p<0.05). The former recorded a mean of 3.8 distressing

Table 6.2 Most distressing symptoms reported during the premenstruum, by GHQ status

Symptom	% reporting as distressing	% GHQ+ reporting as distressing	% GHQ– reporting as distressing	Yule's Q	Chi square
1 Irritability	38	58	29	+0.55	p<0.02
2 Swelling	24	29	24	+0.14	NS
3 Headaches	22	38	15	+0.56	p<0.02
4 Depression	19	42	9	+0.75	p<0.001
5 Moods	19	21	18	+0.08	NS
6 Weight gain	19	29	15	+0.42	NS
7 Tiredness	18	29	13	+0.48	NS
8 Tension	15	25	11	+0.46	NS
9 Backache	14	17	13	+0.16	NS
10 Tender breasts	14	13	15	–0.09	NS
11 Pain	13	8	15	–0.30	NS
12 Anxiety	11	25	5	+0.70	p<0.02

Source: Scambler and Scambler 1986

Table 6.3 Most distressing symptoms reported during menstrual flow, by GHQ status

Symptom	% reporting as distressing	% GHQ+ reporting as distressing	% GHQ– reporting as distressing	Yule's Q	Chi square
1 Irritability	29	46	22	+0.50	p<0.05
2 Pain	23	21	24	–0.08	NS
3 Tiredness	22	29	18	+0.30	NS
4 Depression	18	29	13	+0.48	NS
5 Moods	18	17	18	–0.05	NS
6 Backache	15	17	15	+0.08	NS
7 Headache	14	21	11	+0.36	NS
8 Swelling	13	13	13	–0.01	NS
9 Weight gain	13	17	11	+0.24	NS
10 Anxiety	11	13	11	+0.07	NS
11 Avoidance of social activity	11	13	11	+0.07	NS
12 Lowered performance	11	17	9	+0.33	NS

Source: Scambler and Scambler 1986

symptoms and the latter a mean of 2.5. Table 6.3 shows, in rank order, the 12 symptoms most frequently defined as distressing during the menstrual flow. Only one of these, irritability, was significantly associated with GHQ+ status. Eight of the remaining 11 symptoms showed a positive but non-significant association with GHQ+ status.

Only 15 per cent of the sample of 79 women recorded one or more distressing symptoms during the remainder of the cycle. More of those with GHQ+ status (25 per cent) did so than those with GHQ– status (11 per cent), but this difference was not statistically significant. Those with GHQ+ status reported a mean of 0.11 distressing symptoms, and those with GHQ– status a mean of 0.08. Only depression (4 per cent), skin disorder (3 per cent) and difficulty sleeping (3 per cent) were defined as distressing by more than 1 per cent of the sample. None of the 34 symptoms on the MMDQ were associated with GHQ+ status at anything like a level of statistical significance.

These data are suggestive in at least two ways. First, they point to possible links between psychiatric symptomatology and menstrual symptom reporting. This appears most marked for the premenstruum, but is discernible also for menstrual flow; it all but disappears for the remainder of the cycle. Second, the difference in menstrual symptom reporting between those displaying and those not displaying psychiatric symptomatology is most obvious in relation to 'psychological' symptoms. Clare (1980) divided 30 of the 34 symptoms on the abbreviated MMDQ into three categories: 'physical' (11), 'psychological' (12) and 'behavioural' (7). Table 6.4 draws on this division to highlight the significance of GHQ status by psychological compared with physical and behavioural symptom reporting.

Table 6.4 GHQ status by mean number of symptoms defined as distressing, by symptom type and by phase of menstrual cycle

	Phase of menstrual cycle Mean number of distressing symptoms					
	Premenstruum		Menstrual flow		Remainder of cycle	
Symptom type	GHQ+	GHQ–	GHQ+	GHQ–	GHQ+	GHQ–
Physical	1.58	1.07	1.29	0.90	0	0.27
Psychological	2.50	1.03	1.79	1.07	0.58	0.25
Behavioural	0.41	0.25	0.46	0.40	0.14	0.14

Source: Scambler and Scambler 1986

Two methodological concerns require addressing. The first concerns the degree of possible overlap between the measures of psychiatric symptomatology (the 30-item GHQ) and menstrual distress (the 34-item MMDQ). Clare (1980), who utilized the same measures, tested extensively for degree of overlap and found it to be minimal. Moreover, he found what overlap there was to be largely irrelevant for findings which, as far as the premenstruum is concerned, were remarkably similar to those presented here. The second has to do with the possibility of women's GHQ scores being affected according to the phase of menstrual cycle in which they were obtained. The authors tested for this and found there to be no significant relationship between the phase of the menstrual cycle the GHQ was completed in and GHQ scores.

How, then, is the apparent relationship between the presence of psychiatric symptomatology and an identifiable pattern of symptom reporting before and during menses to be interpreted (setting aside here the question of the MMDQ's bias towards negative aspects of menstruation)? Scambler and Scambler (1986) mention two rival interpretations without having the data at their disposal to decide between them. It could be that women with psychiatric symptomatology, perhaps rooted in biographical disruption of one kind or another, actually experience more premenstrual or menstrual distress than others. The psychiatric symptomatology might then be of some aetiological significance. Or, alternatively, it could be that women with psychiatric symptomatology are merely more 'sensitized' to premenstrual or menstrual change than others and therefore more likely to identify change in terms of distressing symptoms (Taylor 1979). To use Harris' (1989) phrase, psychiatric symptomatology might have more to do with 'psychic reactivity' than with aetiology.

To summarize, it was shown initially that premenstrual and menstrual change can lead directly or indirectly to biographical disruption, for example through absence from school or work. The question as to whether or not such change was directly implicated in reduced work performance was seen to be controversial, and to raise ideological issues of gender differentiation as well as empirical issues. Problems of coping at school or work likewise provoked discussion of ideological issues. After a comment on sporting activity, the debate about the advantages, disadvantages and implications for women of recent legal decisions affirming the potential for premenstrual change – medically diagnosed as premenstrual syndrome or PMT – to render those experiencing it temporarily not responsible for their actions were discussed.

Finally, it has been suggested that while change associated with the menstruum can cause biographical disruption, so biographical disruption, sometimes predisposing to psychiatric symptomatology, can lead to menstrual change; the relationship is properly regarded as two-way or dialectical. Psychiatric symptomatology may also enhance the probability that women acknowledge premenstrual or menstrual change and define it as a form of illness. More research, especially along the lines of that contributed by Harris (1989), is needed.

Chapter 7

Rethinking menstruation

A wide range of issues have been raised in the preceding six chapters and it is time to take stock. In this final chapter an attempt is made to develop and deploy a new framework within which menstruation, menstrual change and medically defined disorders of the menstruum might better be accommodated. Discussion in the first section is tied to the elucidation of three themes: *cultural patterning, legitimation* and *medicalization*. It is in large measure the function of this discussion to define the substantially unresolved tensions about periods that surface in contemporary western women's own experiences and accounts.

The second section focuses, first, on some of the key political and structural aspects of gender relations in Britain and kindred societies, in terms of which, arguably, many of the outstanding tensions around periods require to be understood and eventually resolved. Second, and to close this volume, special attention is paid to some of the courses of action open to physicians and other health workers committed to the provision of good quality investigative, diagnostic and, especially, therapeutic services for women presenting with menstrual problems.

UNRESOLVED TENSIONS

The three themes to be introduced and pursued here serve a heuristic purpose, that is, they provide a convenient means by which a hetero-geneous assembly of issues might be collated and presented. The first to be explored is cultural patterning.

Cultural patterning

The discussions in chapter 3 and parts of chapter 4 showed that how girls or women perceive and respond to menstruation and menstrual change derives very largely from their reference groups and the culture in which those groups are embedded. In the years preceding menarche, mothers – or occasionally other female kin or peers – are generally the principal agents of socialization in relation to periods and their day-to-day ramifications. This is true independently of what mothers say, or even of whether or not they say anything at all; silence can be every bit as eloquent in the messages it imparts as a rehearsed speech. Moreover, what mothers say about menstruation may in any case not be consistent with how they behave when it occurs. Typically, men – and most importantly fathers – remain uninvolved, compelling testimony in its own right that periods are 'women's business'.

What this early socialization often conveys is that menstruation is the biological 'fate' of women rather than an affirmation of womanhood; and that talk about it and its character and impact should be confined to females and to the private domain. Menstruation, above all else, calls for discretion in male-dominated public arenas. It carries connotations almost of stigma. Girls learn to follow a set of rules, a 'menstrual etiquette' as Laws (1985) calls it, which they are too young to appraise or challenge. Boys, uninvolved, and with their own role models and peer groups, follow a more leisurely, alternative and circuitous route to the same set of rules.

Given the negative aspects of the concept of menstruation absorbed through late childhood and adolescence, it is not surprising that many adult women seem predisposed to associate menstrual change with physical or psychological distress, social handicap, and even illness. At least, such would seem to be the dominant cultural pattern. One might perhaps most appropriately refer to this notion of a dominant cultural pattern as constituting a Weberian ideal type. As made clear earlier in the text, there is no implication either that all girls and women are socialized in this way (i.e. that the dominant cultural pattern identified here is the only one), or that early family-based or secondary socialization is in any sense irreversible.

Legitimation

As chapter 6 bore testimony, menstrual change can be precipitated by psychological or social factors. Such factors also influence and shape women's perceptions of menstrual change, most conspicuously in terms of the dominant cultural pattern – of negativity – identified both here and in numerous other studies. It should go without saying that neither of these findings justifies the inference that menstrual change is somehow unreal. That the reality of menstrual change is in fact still frequently debated, even contested, suggests problems of 'legitimation'. In other words, there is as yet no authoritative and binding social consensus on the concept of menstrual change; rather, there are multiple concepts of change.

One way of proceeding is to adapt a famous line by Thomas and Thomas (1928): 'If women define situations as real, they are real in their consequences'. According to the analytic framework for women's perceptions of menstrual change introduced in chapter 3, women may variously experience and interpret change as indicative of either a positively or, more commonly, a negatively evaluated altered state, only contingently health related; or they may see it as symptomatic of illness, which is of course necessarily health related. Clearly the 'same' menstrual change, measured against other- or publicly-defined criteria, such as 'extent of blood loss', may be differently interpreted by different women. Thus, of two women with the 'same' blood loss, one might interpret it positively, perhaps seeing it as a natural part of the cycle, while the other might interpret it as symptomatic of illness, consult a physician and attract both a diagnosis of menorrhagia and a pharmacological remedy. In its most extreme formulation, what any individual woman interprets as normal for her and, extrapolating, for other women, might, in the light of publicly-defined criteria, turn out to be abnormal, and vice versa.

It is apparent that there are significant variations between individual women's interpretations of menstrual change, as well as between women's and men's in general, and women's and physicians' in particular. Despite this, and despite cultural patterning, we take as our starting point women's own variable definitions of their situations. We believe this stance to be both appropriate and compelling.

Medicalization

In so far as menstrual change has been publicly acknowledged as a real – albeit predominantly negative – phenomenon, worthy of respectful assessment and consideration, this has largely been a function of its enhanced medicalization. In other words, the medical profession's construction of discrete categories of symptom, disorder or disease associated with menstrual change, the most salient of which are amenorrhoea, menorrhagia, dysmenorrhoea and premenstrual syndrome, has afforded a certain legitimacy to women's accounts of menstrual change. But this source of legitimacy has proved far from straightforward.

In chapter 4 it was revealed that even women both predisposed to link menstruation with illness and experiencing high levels of symptom distress were often reluctant to consult or re-consult a physician. According to many, physicians, archetypically but not exclusively male, 'simply do not understand'. In other words, there typically exists what Freidson (1970) calls a 'clash of perspectives' between women and their physicians regarding problems associated with the menstruum. From the women's perspective, physicians, assertively conveying either a narrow biomedical approach to problem-solving or an overt or covert sexism, were inclined to lack comprehension of women's rationale for consulting and empathy for the women themselves. Moreover, the biomedical approach seemed to show a remarkably small return, most conspicuously in terms of the easing of distress.

There is a paradox here. On the one hand, physicians have played an important part in legitimating menstrual change: they now not only accept but proclaim it as real in textbooks and surgeries. Paradigmatically, they have successfully testified in court not only that premenstrual change is real, sometimes warranting a diagnosis of premenstrual syndrome, but that premenstrual syndrome can be an excusing condition even in cases of alleged homicide. On the other hand, there is an unease felt by many women – importantly, not just feminist critics – that goes beyond mere dissatisfaction with the nature of the biomedical perspective, and the effectiveness of clinical interventions. Some women have articulated this unease in terms of the price they are paying for being taken seriously about menstrual change. For example, in the last chapter it was noted that the medical concept of premenstrual syndrome, by sanctioning the taking away of women's responsibility for their actions over several days each month, can be utilized against as well as for women. The various negative implications of legitimation through medicalization are significant enough to require some elaboration here.

GENDER, MEDICINE AND MENSTRUAL CHANGE

That gender has been an influential factor in the social construction of categories of diagnosis and investigative and therapeutic practice in and around the largely man-made institution of modern allopathic medicine should be apparent from the text of chapter 2. But the salience of gender in relation to health and medicine needs to be interpreted in light of the theses that medicine governs access to the 'sick role' and has become an increasingly important agency of social control. What lies behind these claims?

Parsons (1951) defined illness as a form of deviance on the grounds that it disrupts the social system by inhibiting people's performance of their various social roles. If this disruption is to be minimized, then the behaviour associated with illness, which unlike other forms of deviant behaviour cannot be prevented by the threat of sanctions, must be controlled. Control is exercised through the prescription of a social role for the sick. It has been said that physicians serve as gatekeepers, policing access to this 'sick role' by authoritatively determining who is sick and who is healthy. They also spur the urge to leave the sick role. The sick role itself consists of two rights and two obligations. Sick people's rights are exemption from normal social roles and freedom from responsibility for their own state. The obligations are that sick people must want to get well as quickly as possible, and consult and co-operate with physicians when appropriate. Failure to meet either or both of these obligations may lead to the charge that people are responsible for the continuation of their illness, and ultimately to sanctions, including the withdrawal of the rights of the sick role.

While Parsons is uncritical of physicians acting as agents of social control, regarding it as a limited and socially necessary function, Freidson (1970) is among those who are less sanguine. He argues that physicians' social control functions now extend far beyond the policing of the sick role and possess negative as well as positive potential. Often this negative potential is realized through medicalization.

The points we want to make here are general ones. To return to the paradox noted earlier: while the legitimation of menstrual change through medicalization has apparently worked to women's advantage – by affording them easier access to the sick role for menstrual complaints – there are potential costs as well as benefits. The well-documented medicalization of pregnancy and childbirth serves as an exemplar here.

In their comparison of revealingly divergent maternal and medical perspectives on pregnancy, Graham and Oakley (1981) show how physicians have increasingly come to define and respond to pregnancy *as if* it were a form of sickness. In their commentary Doyal and Elston write, 'Medical decision-making is strongly influenced by the view that it is a lesser error to treat a well person as sick than a sick person as well. Applied to pregnancy, this decision-making rule justifies intervention "just in case" ' (1986: 192). Oakley (1980; 1984) has shown just how intrusive and 'controlling' male-dominated obstetrics has become, in relation to antenatal care provided regularly throughout pregnancy as well as to labour and to childbirth; many women experience birth not as a natural or normal process but as a hospitalized and high-tech medical event. Moreover, Tew (1990) has painstakingly undermined physicians' principal justification of the medicalization of childbirth, namely, that it has led to safer childbirth.

This argument is not of course directed against the involvement of physicians in pregnancy and childbirth or the use of hospitals and their technologies *per se*; indeed, these services continue to be of enormous and undisputed benefit to a small minority of women. Rather, it is against what most women with potentially normal, trouble-free pregnancies, labours and births experience as – or as equivalent to– an irrational, extended and enforced occupancy of the sick role, culminating in an active third-party management of the birth process. The costs of medicalization in such cases typically outweigh the benefits.

Menstruation has not yet been medicalized to the extent of pregnancy and childbirth. Again, there is no disputing that there are circumstances in which physicians might appropriately and usefully be consulted and access to the sick role appropriately sanctioned. But, equally, some commentators argue that the costs of the current degree of medicalization of menstrual change already exceed the benefits. There are two key points to make here. First, it is clear that physicians' understanding of the menstrual cycle and definitions of menstrual disorders are open to question. Textbook accounts of menstrual disorders are marked by uncertainty. After reviewing contemporary textbooks, Laws writes, 'These texts appear to have difficulties in the definition of every kind of menstrual problem' (1990: 148). And, marginally less bluntly:

> My overriding impression of the material in gynaecology texts on menstrual problems is that very little is known about them, and that little more is likely to be learnt unless some major change of attitudes comes about for the texts are full of 'let-out clauses' providing excuses for their lack of attention to these problems.
>
> (Laws 1990: 152)

In this same review Laws characterizes the medical textbook perspective in the following terms. Gynaecologists are principally oriented towards the uncovering of diseases; they show a marked reticence in defining normal menstrual phenomena, leaving readers to make their own inferences on the basis of definitions of allegedly abnormal menstrual phenomena; if– and typically only if – organic causes for abnormal phenomena cannot be found, they hypothesize some unidentifiable psychological aetiology; and, while in the absence of organic causes they may or may not advise treating the symptoms physically, they rarely if ever advise psychotherapy ('unless you count pep talks from themselves').

Not surprisingly, textbook uncertainties are mirrored in clinical practice. Thus, for example, when a woman presents with what she perceives to be excessive bleeding, the physician will probably diagnose menorrhagia – generally without attempting to measure the extent of blood loss – and proceed to investigate for organic causes, like uterine fibroids. If no such causes are found, as they are not in approximately half the cases of diagnosed menorrhagia (occasioning references to dysfunctional uterine bleeding), then psychosomatic causation may be imputed. Any therapeutic intervention for dysfunctional uterine bleeding, however, will almost certainly be physical rather than psychological (see chapter 1). Had we focused on amenorrhoea, dysmenorrhoea or, most notoriously of all, premenstrual syndrome here, instead of menorrhagia, the message would have been essentially the same (see Laws 1990). And as argued in chapter 5, physicians' readiness to apply medical labels to poorly defined but allegedly abnormal premenstrual and menstrual change, and hence to sanction access to the sick role, not only constitutes evidence of medicalization but invites reflection on the thesis that medicine is an important agency of social control affecting women in a patriarchal society. Given common findings of surveys utilizing the Moos Menstrual Distress Questionnaire, at least four out of every five menstruating women, it seems, report 'distressing symptoms' of premenstrual or menstrual change (Scambler and Scambler 1985). Many, or even most, of them would qualify for nomination to the sick role.

The second point concerns the social contexts in which this medicalization of menstrual phenomena needs to be interpreted. Laws' view is that, for all the significance of their policing and gatekeeping roles, physicians are followers rather than leaders: 'Gynaecologists act primarily as men, and only secondarily as doctors – their work is a form of mediation between the male culture's view of women and the problems that women seek help with' (1990: 133). Moreover, gender has a marked effect on what Mechanic (1978) terms self- and other-defined 'illness behaviour' in, but also around, the sick role. In other words, gender socialization influences both how women define and react to illness and how accommodating others are. In his study of a pottery factory, Bellaby makes this point in relation to age and class as well as to gender. Employers may have been obliged, he writes, to accept physicians' rulings on access to the sick role, but

> workmates and managers mediated the path to a clinical consultation, and their reaction after sickness was certified did not necessarily endorse the doctor's interpretation, even if that ruling had to be

accepted for sick pay purposes. This expanded context for the sick role is one in which, not the specific and universal requirements of contract, but the diffuse and particular relations of gender, age and class shape the pretexts on which absence through sickness is acceptable.

(1990: 63)

It is apparent that an employer's threshold of accommodation of a female employee's period pains or perceived monthly mood swings might vary in accordance with his need to retain her. During a phase of near full employment for local people with the relevant skills he might be more accommodating than during a phase when replacement employees are plentiful. In the first circumstance he might smooth his employee's path to the sick role for her benefit; and in the second he might smooth her path to the sick role to her cost. The extent to which the medicalization of menstrual change benefits or costs a woman, then, may be contingent upon the social context in which she finds herself at any given time.

And, to recall Martin's (1989) argument from chapter 6, this micro-level analysis has applicability also at the macro-level. Martin suggested that at times of ubiquitous unemployment, when government policies are typically directed at keeping women at home, there tend to be more published studies purporting to demonstrate links between menstrual change, disease and impaired work performance than at times of full employment, when government policies are typically directed at recruiting women (often described in Marx's words as a 'reserve army of labour'). Needless to say, there is as yet a paucity of empirical material available to test out these ideas, either at micro- or macro-level.

We have, then, utilized the familiar and related notions of the sick role and social control to build on the general statements in chapter 2. We emphasize the importance of appreciating that current popular *and medical* concepts of menstruation and menstrual disorders have been socially constructed over time and in evolving and predominantly patriarchal societies. Inevitably they reflect these origins. Health professionals committed to helping women who present with menstrual problems can no longer afford to behave as if medical concepts and practices exist in social and cultural vacuums. But what can they do?

PROVIDING GOOD-QUALITY CARE

It behoves individual practitioners to be aware that social change in patriarchal societies – for example, medicalization in general, and the medicalization of pregnancy and childbirth or of menstrual change in particular – will tend to create new opportunities for affirming gender inequalities. Often, such opportunities will be unintended rather than intended consequences of change. In this sense, and in the parlance of contemporary feminism, health work requires 'engendering': physicians and other health workers need to be aware, as documented in chapter 2, that their textbooks, their practices and, most importantly, the unintended consequences of each, continue to reflect and reproduce inequalities between men and women.

It is in this context that Weideger (1975) refers to 'the gynaecologist as shaman'. She writes,

> The shaman, because of his training, knowledge and role, conserves the values of his society. He works to maintain the beliefs which give his culture shape and reinforces the power of the spirits who guide his people. The shaman cures by showing those who have strayed the way back onto the path of righteousness – unless, of course, they have strayed too far.
>
> (1975: 140).

It is when history-taking and investigations fail to reveal organic causes for menstrual problems, Weideger contends, that gynaecologists typically resort to 'divine guidance'. And this divine guidance tends to take the form of injunctions to conform both to the menstrual taboo or etiquette and to conventional segregated gender roles. Thus:

> Menstruation is the 'badge of femininity'. Whether it is worn in misery, pain or pride depends on a woman's attitude toward herself as a female, and her biologic destiny – marriage and motherhood.
>
> (Kroger 1962: 257)

Laws (1990) has highlighted these same gender stereotypes that occur in recent British gynaecology texts, most notably perhaps in the fourth edition of Sir Norman Jeffcoate's *Principles of Gynaecology* (1975).

Needless to say, the 'engendering' of health work in a patriarchal society is no small task, destined in the short term to be ridiculed and denied by professional spokesmen and outside commentators alike. Moreover, just as the medicalization of menstrual change has costs as well as benefits for women so would a de-medicalization of menstrual change for example, restricted access to the sick role and to professional help.

We argued earlier that, regardless of the likely relevance of cultural patterning, women's own definitions of their situations should be taken as the starting point. What, then, are some of the implications of the material included in this volume for physicians advising women whose definitions of their situations lead them to present with menstrual problems?

A family of three related themes stand out. The first is the *'engendering' of health work*. As was shown in earlier chapters, this task involves far more than combating overt sexism in medical practice. Most fundamentally, it calls for a painstaking and critical reconstitution of both textual medical knowledge and what Lock calls the 'folk models' which for many individual physicians 'form the basis for their decision-making' (1982: 277). This will necessarily entail extending and elaborating upon extant research into the menstrual cycle and disorders associated with it.

The second theme also involves research, this time properly to *evaluate the outcomes of medical interventions for menstrual disorders*. As in many other areas of medicine, such research is as yet in its infancy. Consider, for example, the use of hysterectomies to relieve menstrual disorders. Menorrhagia is in fact the main presenting symptom in approximately 60 per cent of cases. On current rates, at least 20 per cent of women in England and Wales will have a hysterectomy before the age of 65. Moreover, about a third of all uteri removed at hysterectomy are pathologically normal. Coulter summarizes the possible costs and benefits of hysterectomies in cases of menorrhagia as follows:

A woman recommended for hysterectomy, at the average age (in Britain) of 40–45, to relieve symptoms of heavy menstrual bleeding, faces a number of important consequences. On the benefit side, the operation will result in the cessation of menstrual bleeding, thus removing the problem for which she sought help; she will no longer have to worry about contraception; she will no longer run the risk of uterine cancer; and there may be other social and psychological advantages to her. On the cost side, she will have to undergo a major operation with associated risks of mortality, morbidity and complications; she will be unable to carry out her normal activities for a period of time; she will no longer be able to bear children; if her ovaries are removed at the same time, as is sometimes the case, she will undergo an immediate artificial menopause, and she will probably have to undergo a course of hormone replacement therapy with a further set of associated risks; and she may risk other social and psychological complications. Weighing up the risks and benefits of this procedure is, therefore, no easy task, either at the individual level, or at the population level when determining health policy.

(1991: 125)

Reviewing evaluative studies in this area to date, Coulter concludes that 'they present a fragmented and inconclusive picture' (1991: 129).

The final theme concerns physician–patient encounters and the progression to good quality care. Such encounters should not of course only be focused on the efficient and cost-effective biomedical pursuit of disease and its management. Co-participation in menstrual care would ensure that women were listened to, informed and advised rather than interrogated and instructed. Women's own expertise would be acknowledged. Co-participation in care would therefore necessarily entail the abandonment of the – frequently sexist – physician–shaman role. An *open agenda* during consultations about menstrual problems, as opposed to one pre-set and enforced by physicians, would permit women to pose questions arising from their own lay perspectives, as well as responding to those originating in the medical perspective. An open agenda would also take physicians beyond a learned biomedical and towards a *holist* orientation, requiring them to address the reasons underlying women's decisions to consult and the significance of their presenting problems in their lives. Finally, if listening with respect can be intrinsically therapeutic, it would on occasions be possible for physicians to offer more positive *counselling*, utilizing skills developed over many decades by psychologists (and, as yet, largely inaccessible in medical training) (see Scambler 1990).

One additional comment on this third theme ought to be appended here. It might be argued that to propogate such broad extra-biomedical criteria of good quality care is unrealistic given scarce resources, not least consultation time. Our response is that, if the criteria are rational and appropriate, they should not be abandoned because they cannot currently be applied; rather, we should face up to the fact that we are unable to deliver good quality care on existing resources. However commendable, optimum care given existing resources is not necessarily good quality care. In any event, as this volume has illustrated, optimum care for women with self-defined menstrual problems remains to be achieved.

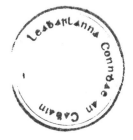

References

CHAPTER ONE

Anderson, A. and McPherson, A. (1983) 'Menstrual problems', in A. Anderson and A. McPherson (eds) *Women's Problems in General Practice*, Oxford: Oxford University Press.

Barnes, J. and Chamberlain, G. (1988) *Lecture Notes on Gynaecology*, 6th edn, Oxford: Blackwell Scientific Publications.

Elder, M. (ed.) (1988) *Reproduction, Obstetrics and Gynaecology*, London: Heinemann.

Frank, R. (1931) 'The hormonal causes of premenstrual tension', *Archives of Neurology and Psychiatry* 26: 1053–7.

Fry, J. (1979) *Common Diseases*, 2nd edn, Lancaster: MTP.

MacKenzie, I. and Bibby, J. (1978) 'Critical assessment of dilatation and curettage in 1029 women', *The Lancet* ii: 566.

Ricci, J. (1950) *The Genealogy of Gynaecology*, Philadelphia: Blakiston.

Richards, D. (1979) 'A general practice view of functional disorders associated with menstruation', *Res. Clin. Forums* 1: 39.

Sanders, D. (1983) 'Premenstrual tension', in A. Anderson and A. McPherson (eds) *Women's Problems in General Practice*, Oxford: Oxford University Press.

Vessey, M., Clarke, J. and MacKenzie, I. (1979) 'Dilatation and curettage in young women', *Health Bulletin*, March: 59.

Vollman, R. (1977) *The Menstrual Cycle*, Philadelphia: W. B. Saunders.

Weideger, P. (1975) *Female Cycles*, London: The Women's Press.

CHAPTER TWO

Allen, I. (1988) *Doctors and their Careers*, London: Policy Studies Institute.

Broverman, K., Broverman, D., Clarkson, F., Rosenkrantz, P. and Vogel, S. (1970), 'Sex role stereotypes and clinical judgement of mental health', *Journal of Consulting and Clinical Psychology* 34: 1–7.

Busfield, J. (1988) 'Mental illness as social product or social construct: a contradiction in feminists' arguments?', *Sociology of Health and Illness* 10: 521–42.

Chesler, P. (1972) *Women and Madness*, New York: Doubleday.

Cooperstock, R. (1981) 'A review of women's psychotropic drug use', in E. Howell and M. Bayes (eds) *Women and Mental Health*, New York: Basic Books.

Department of Health (1991) 'Women doctors and their careers', Report of the Joint Working Party. London: Department of Health.

Down, J. (1867) 'Influence of the sewing-machine on female health', *British Medical Journal* 12, January: 26–7.

Doyal, L. and Elston, M. (1986) 'Women, health and medicine', in V. Beechey and E. Whitelegg, (eds) *Women in Britain Today*, Milton Keynes: Open University Press.

Ehrenreich, B. and English, D. (1974a) *Witches, Midwives and Nurses: a History of Women Healers*, London: Glass Mountain Pamphlet No. 1.

Ehrenreich, B. and English, D. (1974b) *Complaints and Disorders: the Sexual Politics of Sickness*, London: Glass Mountain Pamphlet No. 2.

Ehrenreich, B. and English, D. (1978) 'The "sick" women of the upper classes', in J. Ehrenreich, (ed.) *The Cultural Crisis of Modern Medicine*, New York: Monthly Review Press.

Geddes, P. and Thompson, A. (1890) *The Evolution of Sex*, New York: Scriber & Welford.

Laws, S. (1990) *Issues of Blood: the Politics of Menstruation*, London: Macmillan.

Leeson, J. and Gray, J. (1978) *Women and Medicine*, London: Tavistock Publications.

Martin, E. (1989) *The Woman in the Body: a Cultural Analysis of Reproduction*, Milton Keynes: Open University Press.

Sayers, J. (1982) *Biological Politics: Feminist and Anti-Feminist Perspectives*, London: Tavistock Publications.

Shelvin, B. (1981) 'Painful patients and happy doctors', in G. Edwards (ed.) *Psychiatry in General Practice*, Southampton: Southampton University Press.

Stacey, M. (1988) *The Sociology of Health and Healing*, London: Unwin Hyman.

CHAPTER THREE

AuBuchon, P. and Calhoun, K. (1985) 'Menstrual cycle symptomatology: the role of social expectancy and experimental demand characteristics', *Psychosomatic Medicine* 47: 35–45.

Clark, A. and Ruble, D. (1978) 'Young adolescents' beliefs concerning menstruation', *Child. Dev.* 49: 231–4.

Clare, A. and Wiggins, R. (1979) 'The construction of a modified version of the Menstrual Distress Questionnaire for use in general practice populations', in L. Carenza and L. Zichella (eds) *Emotion and Reproduction*, vol. 20A, London: Academic Press.

Deutsch, H. (1944) *The Psychology of Women*, New York: Grune & Stratton.

Frazer, J. (1959) *The New Golden Bough*, ed. T. Gaster, New York: New American Library.

Greer, G. (1971) *The Female Eunuch*, London: Paladin.

Hays, H. (1972) *The Dangerous Sex*, New York: Pocket Books.

Higgins, P. (1984) 'Things aren't always what they seem', *Journal of the Royal Society of Medicine* 77: 728–37.

Johnson, S. and Snow, L. (1982) 'Assessment of reproductive knowledge in an inner-city clinic', *Social Science and Medicine* 16: 1657–62.

Kessel, N. and Coppen, A. (1963) 'The prevalence of menstrual symptoms', *The Lancet* 2: 61–4.

Moos, R. (1968) 'The development of a menstrual distress questionnaire', *Psychosomatic Medicine* 30: 853–67.

Moos, R. (1969) 'A typology of menstrual cycle symptoms', *American Journal of Obstetrics and Gynecology* 103: 390–402.

Moos, R. (1977) *Menstrual Distress Manual*, Palo Alto: Social Ecology Laboratory.

Novak, E. (1921) *Menstruation and its Disorders*, New York: Appleton & Co.

Olasov, B. and Jackson, J. (1987) 'Effects of expectancies on women's reports of moods during the menstrual cycle', *Psychosomatic Medicine* 49: 65–78.

Parlee, M. (1974) 'Stereotypic beliefs about menstruation: a methodological note on the Moos menstrual distress questionnaire and some new data', *Psychosomatic Medicine* 36: 229–40.

Scambler, A. and Scambler, G. (1985) 'Menstrual symptoms, attitudes and consulting behaviour', *Social Science and Medicine* 20: 1065–8.

Shainess, N. (1961) 'A re-evaluation of some aspects of femininity through a study of menstruation', *Comparative Psychiatry* 2: 20–6.

Skultans, V. (1970) 'The symbolic significance of menstruation and the menopause', *Man* 5: 639–51.

Snow, L. and Johnson, S. (1977) 'Modern day menstrual folklore: some clinical implications', *Journal of the American Medical Association* 237: 2736–9.

Weideger, P. (1975) *Female Cycles*, London: The Women's Press.

Whisnant, L. and Zegans, L. (1965) 'A study of attitudes toward menarche in white middle-class American girls', *American Journal of Psychiatry* 132: 809–14.

Woods, N., Kramer Dery, G. and Most, A. (1982) 'Recollections of menarche, current menstrual attitudes and perimenstrual symptoms', *Psychosomatic Medicine* 44: 285–93.

CHAPTER FOUR

Cartwright, A. and Anderson, R. (1981) *General Practice Revisited: a Second Study of Patients and their Doctors*, London: Tavistock Publications.

Freidson, E. (1970) *Profession of Medicine: a Study of the Sociology of Applied Knowledge*, New York: Russell Sage Foundation.

Hannay, D. (1980) 'The iceberg of illness and trivial consultations', *Journal of the Royal College of General Practitioners* 30: 551–4.

Ingham, J. and Miller, P. (1979) 'Symptom prevalence and severity in a general practice', *Journal of Epidemiology and Community Health* 33: 191–8.

Kleinman, A. (1985) 'Indigenous systems of healing: questions for professional, popular, and folk care', in J. Salmon (ed.) *Alternative Medicines: Popular and Policy Perspectives*, London: Tavistock Publications.

Last, J. (1963) 'The iceberg: completing the clinical picture in general practice', *The Lancet* 2: 28–31.

Roberts, H. (1985) *The Patient Patients: Women and their Doctors*, London: Pandora.

Scambler, A. (1980) 'Women, menstruation and primary care', Unpublished paper presented at staff–postgraduate seminar, Department of General Practice, Guy's Hospital Medical School, London.

Scambler, A., Scambler, G. and Craig, D. (1981) 'Kinship and friendship networks and women's demand for primary care', *Journal of the Royal College of General Practitioners* 26: 746–50.

Scambler, A. and Scambler, G. (1985) 'Menstrual symptoms, attitudes and consulting behaviour', *Social Science and Medicine* 20: 1065–8.

Scambler, G. and Scambler, A. (1984) 'The illness iceberg and aspects of consulting behaviour', in R. Fitzpatrick, J. Hinton, S. Newman, G. Scambler and J. Thompson (eds) *The Experience of Illness*, London: Tavistock Publications.

Schneider, J. and Conrad, P. (1980) 'In the closet with illness: epilepsy, stigma potential and information control', *Social Problems* 28: 32–44.

Suchman, E. (1965) 'Stages of illness and medical care', *Journal of Health and Social Behaviour* 6: 114–28.

Westcott, P. (1987) *Alternative Health Care for Women*, London: Guild Publishing.

Young, G. (1981) 'A woman in medicine: reflections from the inside', in H. Roberts (ed.) *Women, Health and Reproduction*, London: Routledge.

Zola, I. (1973) 'Pathways to the doctor: from person to patient', *Social Science and Medicine* 7: 677–89.

CHAPTER FIVE

Baines, G. and Slade, P. (1988) 'Attributional patterns, moods and the menstrual cycle', *Psychosomatic Medicine* 50: 469–76.

Dalton, K. (1964) *The Premenstrual Syndrome*, London: Heinemann.

Dalton, K. (1969) *The Menstrual Cycle*, Harmondsworth: Penguin Books.

Dalton, K. (1978) *Once a Month*, London: Fontana.

Daly, M. (1978) *Gyn/Ecology*, Boston: Beacon Press.

Hilbourne, J. (1973) 'On disabling the normal: the implications of physical disability for other people', *British Journal of Social Work* 3: 497–507.

Hopson, J. and Rosenfeld, A. (1984) 'PMS: puzzling monthly symptoms', *Psychology Today*, August: 30–5.

Laws, S. (1985a) 'Male power and menstrual etiquette', in H. Thomas (ed.) *The Sexual Politics of Reproduction*, London: Gower.

Laws, S. (1985b) 'Who needs PMT? A feminist approach to the politics of premenstrual tension', in S. Laws, V. Hey and A. Eagan *Seeing Red: the Politics of Pre-menstrual Tension*, London: Hutchinson.

Lever, J. (1980) *PMT: the Unrecognized Illness*, London: New English Library.

Mansfield, P., Hood, K. and Henderson, J. (1989) 'Women and their husbands: mood and arousal fluctuations across the menstrual cycle and days of the week', *Psychosomatic Medicine* 51: 66–80.

Paige, K. (1973) 'Women learn to sing the menstrual blues', *Psychology Today*, September.

Scambler, G. and Scambler, A. (1986) 'Minor psychiatric morbidity and menstruation', *International Journal of Social Psychiatry* 6: 9–15.

Schneider, J. and Conrad, P. (1981) 'Medical and sociological typologies: the case of epilepsy', *Social Science and Medicine* 15A: 211–19.
Shader, P. and Ohly, J. (1970) 'Premenstrual tension, femininity and sexual drive', *Medical Aspects of Human Sexuality*, April: 48.
Shuttle, P. and Redgrove, P. (1980) *The Wise Wound: Menstruation and Everywoman*, Harmondsworth: Penguin Books.
Steinem, G. (1984) 'If men could menstruate', in *Outrageous Acts and Everyday Rebellions*, London: Fontana.
Taylor, D. (1988) *Red Flower: Rethinking Menstruation*, Freedom, Calif.: The Crossing Press.
Weideger, P. (1975) *Female Cycles*, London: The Women's Press.

CHAPTER SIX

Allen, H. (1990) 'At the mercy of her hormones: premenstrual tension and the law', in P. Adams and E. Cowie (eds) *The Woman in Question*, London: Verso.
Andersch, B. and Milsom, I. (1982) 'An epidemiological study of adolescent dysmenorrhoea', *American Journal of Obstetrics and Gynecology* 144: 655–60.
Bass, F. (1947) 'L'amenorrhe au camp de concentration de Terezin', *Gynaecologia* 123: 211–19.
Clare, A. (1980) 'Psychiatric and social aspects of premenstrual complaint', *Psychological Medicine Monograph*, Supplement 4.
Dalton, K. (1960) 'Schoolgirls' behaviour and menstruation', *British Medical Journal* 2: 1647.
Dalton, K. (1968) 'Menstruation and examinations', *The Lancet*, December 28: 1386.
Dalton, K. (1978) *Once a Month*, London: Fontana.
Dalton, K. (1982) 'Legal implications of premenstrual syndrome', *World Medicine*, April 17: 93–4.
Foucault, M. (1979) *Discipline and Punish: the Birth of the Prison*, New York: Vintage.
Frank, R. (1931) 'The hormonal causes of premenstrual tension', *Archives of Neurology and Psychiatry* 26: 1053–7.
Goldberg, D. (1972) *The Detection of Psychiatric Illness by Questionnaire*, Maudsley Monograph No. 21, London: Oxford University Press.
Goldberg, D. and Huxley, P. (1980) *Mental Illness in the Community: The Pathways to Psychiatric Care*, London: Tavistock Publications.
Goldberg, D., Kay, C. and Thompson, L. (1976) 'Psychiatric morbidity in general practice and the community', *Psychological Medicine* 6: 565–9.
Golub, S. (1976) 'The effect of premenstrual anxiety and depression on cognitive function', *Journal of Personality and Social Psychology* 34: 99–104.
Harris, T. (1989) 'Disorders of menstruation', in G. Brown and T. Harris (eds) *Life Events and Illness*, London: Unwin Hyman.
Laws, S. (1985) 'Who needs PMT? A feminist approach to the politics of premenstrual tension', in S. Laws, V. Hey and A. Eagan *Seeing Red: the Politics of Pre-menstrual Tension*, London: Hutchinson.

Laws, S. (1990) *Issues of Blood: the Politics of Menstruation*, London: Macmillan.
Lever, J. (1980) *PMT: the Unrecognized Illness*, London: New English Library.
Martin, E. (1989) *The Woman in the Body: a Cultural Analysis of Reproduction*, Milton Keynes: Open University Press.
Parlee, M. (1973) 'The premenstrual syndrome', *Psychological Bulletin* 80: 454–65.
Scambler, G. and Scambler, A. (1986) 'Minor psychiatric morbidity and menstruation', *International Journal of Social Psychiatry* 6: 9–15.
Shanan, J., Brzezinski, A., Sulman, F. and Sharon, M. (1965) 'Active coping behaviour, anxiety and cortical steroid excretion in the prediction of transient amenorrhoea', *Behavioural Sciences* 10: 461–5.
Shapiro-Peel, N. (1984) 'Resistance strategies: the routine struggle for bread and roses', in K. Brodkin Sacks and D. Remy (eds) *My Troubles are Going to Have Trouble with Me: Everyday Trials and Triumphs of Women Workers*, New Brunswick, NJ: Rutgers University Press.
Squire, C. (1981) 'Indescribable tension', *The Leveller*, 11 December: 16.
Steinem, G. (1984) 'If men could menstruate', in *Outrageous Acts and Everyday Rebellions*, London: Fontana.
Sydenham, A. (1946) 'Amenorrhoea at Stanley Camp, Hong Kong, during internment, *British Medical Journal* 2: 159–60.
Taylor, J. (1979) 'The timing of menstruation-related symptoms assessed by a daily symptom rating scale', *Acta Psychiatrica Scandinavica* 60: 87–105.
Teperi, J. and Rimpela, M. (1989) 'Menstrual pain, health and behaviour in girls', *Social Science and Medicine* 29: 163–9.
Wells, C. (1985) *Women, Sport and Performance: a Physiological Perspective*, Champaign, Ill.: Human Kinetcis Publishing Inc.
Ylikorkala, O. and Dawood, M. (1978) 'New concepts in dysmenorrhoea', *American Journal of Obstetrics and Gynaecology* 130: 833.

CHAPTER SEVEN

Bellaby, P. (1990) 'What is genuine sickness? The relation between work-discipline and the sick role in a pottery factory', *Sociology of Health and Illness* 12: 47–68.
Coulter, A. (1991) 'Evaluating the outcomes of health care', in J. Gabe, M. Calnan and M. Bury (eds) *The Sociology of the National Health Service*, London: Routledge.
Doyal, L. and Elston, M. (1986) 'Women, health and medicine', in V. Beechey and E. Whitelegg (eds) *Women in Britain Today*, Milton Keynes: Open University Press.
Freidson, E. (1970) *The Profession of Medicine: a Study of the Sociology of Applied Knowledge*, New York: Russell Sage Foundation.
Graham, H. and Oakley, A. (1981) 'Competing ideologies of reproduction: medical and maternal perspectives on pregnancy', in H. Roberts (ed.) *Women, Health and Reproduction*, London: Routledge & Kegan Paul.
Jeffcoate, N. (1975) *Principles of Gynaecology*, 4th edn, London: Butterworths.
Kroger, W. (1962) *Psychosomatic Obstetrics, Gynecology and Endocrinology*, Springfield, Ill.: Charles C. Thomas.

Laws, S. (1985) 'Male power and menstrual etiquette', in H. Thomas (ed.) *The Sexual Politics of Reproduction*, London: Gower.

Laws, S. (1990) *Issues of Blood: the Politics of Menstruation*, London, Macmillan.

Lock, M. (1982) 'Models and practice in medicine: menopause as syndrome or life transition?' *Cult. Med. Psychiatr.* 6: 277.

Martin, E. (1989) *The Woman in the Body: a Cultural Analysis of Reproduction*, Milton Keynes: Open University Press.

Mechanic, D. (1978) *Medical Sociology*, 2nd edn, New York: Free Press.

Oakley, A. (1980) *Women Confined*, Oxford: Martin Robertson.

Oakley, A. (1984) *The Captured Womb*, Oxford: Blackwell.

Parsons, T. (1951) *The Social System*, Glencoe: Free Press.

Scambler, A. and Scambler, G. (1985) 'Menstrual symptoms, attitudes and consulting behaviour', *Social Science and Medicine* 20: 1065–8.

Scambler, G. (1990) 'Social factors and quality of life and quality of care in epilepsy', in D. Chadwick (ed.) *Quality of Life and Quality of Care in Epilepsy*, London: Royal Society of Medicine.

Tew, M. (1990) *Safer Childbirth: a Critical History of Maternity Care*, London: Chapman & Hall.

Thomas, W. and Thomas, D. (1928) *The Child in America*, New York: Alfred A. Knopf.

Weideger, P. (1975) *Female Cycles*, London: The Women's Press.

Name index

Allen, H. 80–2
Anderson, A. 6, 7, 12
Anderson, R. 52
AuBuchon, P. 36–7

Baines, G. 62
Barnes, J. 8–9
Bass, F. 83
Bellaby, P. 96–7
Blackwell, Elizabeth 15
Broverman, K. 20
Busfield, J. 19–20

Calhoun, K. 36–7
Cartwright, A. 52
Chamberlain, G. 8–9
Chesler, P. 19
Clare, A. 35, 87–8
Clark, A. 30
Conrad, P. 58
Coppen, A. 33–5
Coulter, A. 99–100

Dalton, Katharina 60–1, 73–6, 79, 80, 82–3
Daly, M. 64
Dawood, M. 73
Deutsch, H. 30
Down, J. 16–18
Doyal, L. 18, 94

Ehrenreich, B. 13, 16, 18, 19
Elder, M. 5, 10, 11
Ellis, 22

Elston, M. 18, 94
English, Christine 80–1
English, D. 13, 16, 18, 19

Foucault, M. 76
Frank, R. 9, 33, 75
Frazer, J. 27
Freidson, E. 47, 93, 94
Fry, J. 11

Garrett Anderson, Elizabeth 15
Geddes, P. 22
Goldberg, D. 85
Graham, H. 94
Gray, J. 16, 18
Greer, G. 30

Hannay, D. 51–2
Harris, T. 83–4, 88–9
Hays, H. 26–7
Heape, 22
Higgins, P. 39
Hilbourne, J. 62
Hopson, J. 56

Jackson, J. 37
Jeffcoate, Norman 98
Johnson, S. 27–9

Kessel, N. 33–5
Kleinman, A. 41, 47
Kroger, W. 98

Last, J. 45

Laws, S. 24, 57–8, 60–1, 63–9, 76, 78, 81–2, 91, 95, 96, 98
Leeson, J. 16, 18
Lever, J. 57, 61, 74–5
Lock, M. 99

McPherson, A. 6, 7, 12
Martin, E. 21–3, 75–8, 97
Mechanic, D. 96
Moebius, 19
Moos, R. 35–6

Oakley, A. 94
Ohly, J. 57
Olasov, B. 37

Paige, K. 65–6
Parlee, M. 36
Parsons, T. 94

Redgrove, P. 61
Richards, D. 11
Rimpella, M. 70–3
Rosenfeld, A. 56
Ruble, D. 30

Sayers, J. 24, 25
Scambler, A. 31, 35, 38, 41, 48, 49–52, 55, 61, 66, 85, 88
Scambler, G. 31, 35, 38, 41, 49–52, 58, 61, 66, 85, 88
Schneider, J. 58
Shader, P. 57
Shanan, J. 84

Shelvin, B. 15–16
Shuttle, P. 61
Skultans, V. 29
Slade, P. 62
Smith, Sandie 80–1
Snow, L. 27–9
Squire, C. 80, 82
Steinem, Gloria 69, 83
Suchman, E. 47–8
Sydenham, A. 83

Taylor, D. 56, 60, 61, 63
Teperi, J. 70–3
Tew, M. 95
Thomas, D. 92
Thomas, W. 92
Thompson, A. 22
Thorburn, J. 18–19

Vessey, M. 8

Weideger, P. 6, 26, 31, 39, 56, 65, 98
Wells, C. 79
Westcott, P. 45–7
Whisnant, L. 30
Wiggins, R. 35
Woods, N. 30–1, 33

Ylikorkala, O. 73
Young, G. 52

Zegans, L. 30
Zola, I. 49

Subject index

Note: Page references in italics indicate tables and figures.

absenteeism: school 71–3, *71, 72, 82*;
    work 73–4, 82
amenorrhoea 5–7, 11; apparent
    (cryptomenorrhoea) 5; causes 83;
    primary 5–7; secondary 5–7;
    83–4; treatment 16, 46
anxiety, as premenstrual symptom
    33, *34*, 60, 85
asthma 774
athletes *see* sport, and menses
attitudes to menstruation: accepting
    31–2, 43, 50; antipathetic 32–3,
    42, 50–1; changing 26–30; and
    experience 31, 32–3, 44–5;
    fatalistic 32, 43, 50–1, 91;
    negative 22–4, 30–3, 37–8, 56,
    62, 77–8, 91; positive 31–2, 37–8,
    39, 56

blood loss 2; assessment 12, 84, 92,
    96; dysfunctional uterine bleeding
    7–8, 11, 96; variations 2–3, *4*, 7, 12
breast tenderness, as premenstrual
    symptom 10, 11, *34*, 56

cancer, endometrial 8
care, co-participation in 100
change, menstrual: impact of
    significant life events 6, 7, 83–9;
    impact on work 70–7;
    legitimation problems 91–2, 93,
    94; male attitudes to 57–62;

medicalization 56, 58, 62, 82, 91,
    92–3, 94–8; and sport 79–80; *see
    also* menstruation
childbirth, medicalization 94–5, 97–8
class: and help-seeking 50–1; and
    medical attitudes to women 16,
    18; and menstrual sex 66
cleanliness, associated with
    menstruation 28
concealment of menstruation 30, 44,
    67–8, 77–8, 91
contagion of menstruation 26–7
contraceptive, intra-uterine: as a
    cause of dysmenorrhoea 9; as
    cause of menorraghia 7
contraceptive, oral: and amenorrhoea
    6; and athletic performance 79;
    and menstrual distress 35
control, social, role of medicine 93–7
corpus albicans 2
corpus luteum 2
counselling 100
crime, and premenstrual syndrome
    80–1, 82
cryptomenorrheoa *see* amenorrhoea,
    apparent
culture: male, and menstruation 63–7,
    68–9, 78, 81, 96; *see also*
    patterning, cultural
curettage *see* D and C

D and C: in treatment of

dysmenorrhoea 9; in treatment of menorraghia 8
definition problems 95
depression: as premenstrual symptom 10, 33, *34*, 56, 60, 85–7; treatments 47
determinism, biological 21–5
deviance, female: illness as 94; medicalization 82–3
diet: and menstrual disorders 6, 46–7; in premenstrual tension 11, 47
discipline, intolerance of 76–7
disease *see* change, menstrual, medicalization
disease/illness distinction 12, 38–9, 45, 53, 88
disorders: evaluation of treatment 99; self-help measures 47; *see also* amenorrhoea, dysmenorrhoea, menorrhagia, premenstrual syndrome
domination, male 57–60, 62, 63–4, 68–9
dysmenorrhoea 7–9, 11, 73, 82; causes 8–9; effects 74; membranous 9; primary 8; secondary 9; treatment 9, 16, 47; *see also* pain

endometriosis 9
endometrium, and ovulation 2, 23
epimenorrhoea 7
etiquette of menstruation 57–8, 63–4, 67–9, 78, 91, 98

fibroid, uterine: as cause of dysmenorrhoea 9; as cause of menorraghia 7–8, 96
folklore, and menstruation 28–9
follicles, Graafian 2
frailty, assumed, of women 16, 18, 19

gender: and medical models of menstruation 21–5, 93–8; in medical perspective 13–20; and social attitudes to menstruation 82–3
General Health Questionnaire 85–8, *87*

headache: as premenstrual symptom 10, 33, *34*, 57, 74, 85; treatments 47
health care system *46*; engendering 98, 99; folk arena 46–7, 49; popular arena 45–7; professional arena 48–51, 98, women's attitudes to 50–2
holist approach 100
hormone: follicle stimulating (FSH) 2; luteinizing (LH) 2; therapy 9, 60–1, 72, 83; *see also* oestrogen; progesterone
hymen, imperforate 5
hypothalamus, role in menstrual cycle 2
hysterectomy: as treatment of dysmenorrhoea 9; as treatment of fibroids 8; as treatment of menorrhagia 99

ignorance, perceived 53
illness: as deviance 94; and help-seeking 45–9, 50–1; menstruation as 41–3, 44, 50–1, 91–3; *see also* disease/illness distinction
inequalities, gender 97–8
instability, perceived female 81–2
intercourse, sexual, during menstruation 29, 44, 64–6, 68
irrationality, and medicalization of menstruation 24, 82
irritability: men's perceptions 66–7; as premenstrual symptom 10, 33, *34*, 55–61, 63, 74–5, 85, 87; treatments 47, 60–1; women's perceptions 55–7
isolation, of menstruating women 26–7

judgement, effects of menstruation on 74–5

language, male 64–5, 66–7
libido, increases 82–3
life events, effects on menstrual change 6, 7, 83–9

medication, for menstrual pain 72–3, *72*

medicine: and patriarchal treatment
of women 13–21, 53, 60, 62; as
socially constructed 13, 23, 58,
93–4, 97; women's perceptions of
50–4, 93
men: attitude to menstruation 36, 37,
63–7, 68–9, 81, 91, 96; attitude to
premenstrual symptoms 55–6,
57–62; 'men's talk' 64–5, 66–7,
78; physicians as 96; relationships
with 55–69
menarche: average age 1; critical
weight 1, 6; delayed 6; as *rite de
passage* 44, 55; women's attitudes
to 30–1, 44
menopause: premature 6; and
treatment of fibroids 7–8
menorrhagia 7–8, 9, 11–12, 82, 92;
causes 7, 83–4, 96; diagnosis 96;
treatments 7–8, 46–7, 99
menstrual cycle 2, *3*; lack of
understanding of 27–9, *28*;
variations in blood loss 2–3, *4*, 7,
12; variations in length 2, 3–5, *4*
menstrual distress score 35
menstrual flow distress score 35
menstruation: as altered state 39, 50,
55, 92; medicalization 21–5, 26,
82, 95–8; seen as disabling 18–19,
91; women's perceptions 26–39,
40; see also attitudes to menstruation
mental disorder, patriarchal
construction 19–21
metrorrhagia 7
mood change *see* irritability
Moos Menstrual Distress
Questionnaire (MMDQ) 35–6, 38,
41, 44, 50, 56, 62, 85–8, 96
mothers, role in socialization 30, 55,
91
myomectomy, as treatment of
fibroids 8

networks, lay referral 47–9, *48*, 50, 54
normality/abnormality: medical
construction 5, 19, 24–5, 26, 95;
social construction 25, 30, 36–8,
41, 44–5, 55–6; women's
perceptions 5, 26–40

oestrogen: in dysmenorrhoea 9; and
premenstrual syndrome 10; role in
menstrual cycle 1–2, 22–3
oligomenorrhoea 6
ovulation 2, *3*

pain 33–6, *34*, 63; adolescent girls
70–3, *71*, *72*; seen as excuse 66;
use of medication 71–3, *72; see
also* dysmenorrhoea
patriarchy: and attitudes to
menstruation 63, 79, 93, 97; in
medicine 13–19, 23–4, 26, 53, 62,
82, 96, 98; and psychiatry 19–21;
see also domination, male
patterning, cultural 90–1, 98; *see also*
socialization
pelvic inflammatory disease 9
performance *34*; academic 73;
sporting 79–80; work 74–7, 88, 97
physicians: male/female 52–3, 93;
reluctance to consult 28, 51, 52, 53
pituitary gland, role in menstrual
cycle 2, 6
PMT *see* premenstrual syndrome
polymenorrhoea 7
pregnancy, medicalization 94–5, 97–8
premenstrual distress score 35
premenstrual syndrome 9–11, *10*,
33–5; alternative treatment 47;
effects 7; and legal responsibility
80–3, 88, 93; male perceptions
57–62; medical perceptions 58–60,
93; and perceived instability
81–2; and sexual equality 81–2;
symptoms 10, *10*, *59*, 60, 85–7,
86, *87*; treatments 11, 60–1;
women's understanding 55–63
progesterone: and premenstrual
syndrome 10, 61, 76; role in
menstrual cycle 2, 22–3
psychiatry, patriarchy in 19–21
puberty 1–2
pyridoxine, deficiency 11

quality of life, effects on 43–5, 50–1,
66

referral: attitudes to 50–4, 93;

incongruous 51–2; lay networks 47–9, *48*, 50, 54
research, need for 54, 89, 99–100
responsibility, legal 80–3, 88, 93

school: coping with menstruation at 77–9, 88; impact of menstrual pain on attendance 71–3, *71*, *72*
science, as socially constructed 13, 23, 58
sex, and menstruation 29, 44, 64–6, 68
sexism *see* patriarchy
sexualization of menstruation 68
sick role 18, 94–7, 98
skin disorder, as premenstrual symptom 56, 87
sleep problems, as premenstrual symptom 57, 87
socialization: and attitudes to menstruation 25, 36–8, 41, 44–5, 56, 58, 62, 77, 96; role of mothers 30, 55, 91
sport, and menses 73, 79–80, 84, 88
stereotypes, cultural 19, 36, 38, 44, 60, 63, 98
swelling, bodily, as premenstrual symptom 10–11, 33, *34*, 56–7
symptoms: and attitudes to menstruation 31, 32–3, 44–5; medical perspective 38–40; men's

attitudes 36, 37; of premenstrual syndrome 10, *10*, *59*, 62, 85–7, *86*, *87*; psychiatric 84–9; severity and help-seeking 45; women's experience 33–8, *34*, 92–3

taboo, menstrual: in ethnic subcultures 27–30; in traditional cultures 26–7; in western culture 30–3, 44, 63, 98
tension, as premenstrual symptom 33, *34*, 36
thyroid gland, role in menstrual disorders 6, 7

uncertainty, and medicalization of menstruation 24, 95–6

weight, critical 1, 6
weight gain, as premenstrual symptom *34*
well-being, enhanced 56
women: medical attitudes to 16–19; perceptions of medical profession 50–4; role in health care 13–15, *14*, 18, 19, 21, 24; and work 24, 70–9, 97; *see also* gender
work: coping with menstruation at 78–9, 88; and perceived instability 81–2; women at 24, 70–9, 97